LUPUS:
IT CHOSE ME

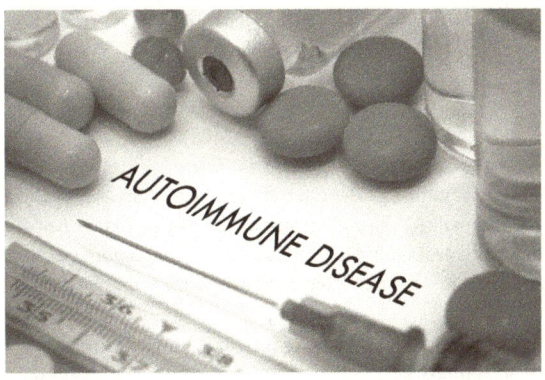

A Walk through the Life of
Autoimmune Disease

LaTonya Bias, PhD

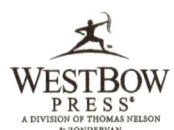

Copyright © 2020 LaTonya Bias, PhD.

All rights reserved. No part of this book may be used or reproduced by any means, graphic, electronic, or mechanical, including photocopying, recording, taping or by any information storage retrieval system without the written permission of the author except in the case of brief quotations embodied in critical articles and reviews.

This book is a work of non-fiction. Unless otherwise noted, the author and the publisher make no explicit guarantees as to the accuracy of the information contained in this book and in some cases, names of people and places have been altered to protect their privacy.

WestBow Press books may be ordered through booksellers or by contacting:

WestBow Press
A Division of Thomas Nelson & Zondervan
1663 Liberty Drive
Bloomington, IN 47403
www.westbowpress.com
1 (866) 928-1240

Because of the dynamic nature of the Internet, any web addresses or links contained in this book may have changed since publication and may no longer be valid. The views expressed in this work are solely those of the author and do not necessarily reflect the views of the publisher, and the publisher hereby disclaims any responsibility for them.

Any people depicted in stock imagery provided by Getty Images are models, and such images are being used for illustrative purposes only.
Certain stock imagery © Getty Images.

Author Credits: Author, CEO of Love Life Lupus Foundation
INC, and Advocate for helping people

THE HOLY BIBLE, NEW INTERNATIONAL VERSION®, NIV® Copyright © 1973, 1978, 1984, 2011 by Biblica, Inc.® Used by permission. All rights reserved worldwide.

Scripture quotations marked (NLT) are taken from the Holy Bible, New Living Translation, copyright © 1996, 2004, 2007 by Tyndale House Foundation. Used by permission of Tyndale House Publishers, Inc., Carol Stream, Illinois 60188. All rights reserved.

ISBN: 978-1-9736-8534-0 (sc)
ISBN: 978-1-9736-8535-7 (hc)
ISBN: 978-1-9736-8533-3 (e)

Library of Congress Control Number: 2020902462

Print information available on the last page.

WestBow Press rev. date: 4/28/2020

One of the lessons I grew up with was to always stay true to yourself and never let what somebody says distract you from your goals.

-Michelle Obama
Former First Lady

Do you not know that your bodies are temples of the Holy Spirit, who is in you, whom you have received from God? You are not your own; you were bought at a price. Therefore, honor God with your bodies.

1 Corinthians 6: 19-20

AN APPRECIATION

I am indebted to God; my husband, children, grandchildren, parents, family, friends, and church members. Thank you all for your understanding and prayers. To my grandmother that loved me unconditionally, may she rest in peace. She was truly remarkable, and I am deeply grateful for the time we spent together.

INTRODUCTION

As a young adult, the Serenity Prayer was provided to me by a family member to help me get through my hard times. I was not addicted, nor did I take drugs or drink alcohol, however, as the Serenity Prayer provided positive motivation towards a foreseeable future. I use the Serenity Prayer to keep me on track in life. Now, I am not saying that the Serenity Prayer can work for everyone; but it worked for me daily. You should try it! When you do, take a breather and close your eyes. Think about something positive and take it slow. Allow your mind to sink into your chest and pray.

SERENITY PRAYER

God, grant me the serenity to accept the things I cannot change, courage to change the things I can, and the wisdom to know the difference …

—Reinhold Niebuhr

LUPUS AWARENESS
SUPPORTING THE FIGHT

It is time, at last, to speak the truth about lupus as I know it. TRUTH IS, after 30 years of ups and downs with this disease, no one knows much about the autoimmune disease called "Lupus". If they did, why are so many people being misdiagnosed? Could new blood be the cure?

To live by medicine is to live horribly

- Carl Linnabus (1707-1778)

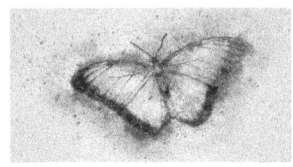

ACKNOWLEDGMENTS

Are you ready to get to the meat of this book? Me too, but first I would like to thank God for waking me up every day and guiding my steps. I would like to thank the love of my life my husband, for providing support and understanding with my illness. Spending long hours in the hospital, being around for every tear, picking up all the responsibility when I have flares, and loving me unconditionally. I want to thank my children (Ki-Ki, Jay, and James) for understanding and keeping me uplifted when I am down, for dancing, singing, and staying strong when I am weak.

Thanks to my grandchildren (Goo-Goo, Nuuk-Nuuk, Man-Man and Gunnar). I enjoy watching their beautiful smiles and hearing their laughter as they grow and enjoy life. I want to thank my Kelli-Wellie and my Jada Bug for bringing bliss into my life. I want to thank my family, whom I love. I cannot name them all: Mom, Dad, my Nana (RIP), all my siblings (Nikki), aunts, uncles, cousins, best and close friends and friends for being my support system.

In the morning, present yourselves, tribe by tribe. The tribe the LORD chooses shall come forward clan by clan; the clan the LORD chooses shall come forward family by family, and the family the LORD chooses shall come forward man by man.

- Joshua 7:14

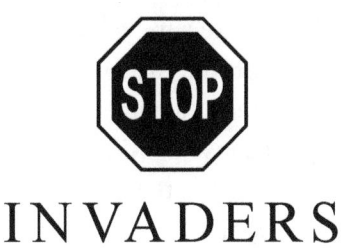

INVADERS

RECEIVING A DIAGNOSIS of lupus is overwhelming. My life has not been the same. Never did I think I would be writing about something so detrimental. My immune system has limitations between outside conditions and indoor environments. I should be living in a bubble. Let me explain why.

When bacteria lands on my skin, part of what keeps the germs from infecting my body is the bodily structure of my epidermis. The epidermis is the outermost layer of our skin; the main purpose is protection. Why am I talking about this? Well, one reason, it forms a boundary between the bacteria and the external environment of homes, schools, and buildings. Two, this is how lupus begins for me; With bacteria! Below are a few tips you should know to help you have fewer invaders (bacteria):

- As soon as you feel like you must go to the restroom, then go. Do Not Hold It! If you find that you have not gone to the restroom all day, make yourself GO. Holding urine too long is not good for your urinary tract system. It can lead to accidents.
- When you go into a restroom make sure, you use your elbow or foot to open the door.
- When you open the door, retrieve a paper towel. If the restroom does not have paper towels or something to dry your hands-LEAVE!
- Use paper towels to open the stall door. If you are in someone's home, use a paper towel to open the door.
- Do not sit on toilets, if you must, thoroughly, place the tissue on the seat.

- When you are done make sure you clean yourself from front to back. Try to tap off all the urine before going behind, not too close to the vaginal area and wipe from front to back. Especially after going poop. Because of where the urethra is, it's easy for bacteria from poop to get in that area causing UTI (urinary tract infections). Most people do not understand that if you clean yourself incorrectly and allow the invaders to get into your vaginal area causing an infection. Carry wet wipes if you can.
- When it's time to flush the toilet use the paper towel to touch the handle.
- When leaving out of the stall use a paper towel to open the door.
- When washing your hands, get a fresh paper towel, use it to turn the faucet on and get your soap. When you are done, use the paper towel to turn the water off, open the door to leave the bathroom.

It is very important to do these steps because you have plenty of microorganisms in the restrooms, including both familiar and unfamiliar such as streptococcus, staphylococcus, E. coli, shigella bacteria, hepatitis A, cold, and various sexually transmitted organisms.

When I breathe in bacteria or toxins through my nose the tiny hairs inside my nose and cilia inside my lungs act as a somatic wall to stop the invaders. At the same time, my immune system builds a chemical blockade, creating a discharge in my nose and lungs that traps and neutralizes many invaders. However, in my life, this did not work for me. The invaders which you will hear me talk about in this book will be referred to as bacteria. I am not sure if you have seen masks that say, "It's not me it's you". I find that to be very real. You must wear a mask almost everywhere you go. If you are around a lot of people you need a mask. Concerts, airports, schools, daycares, or even walking outside to get a breath of fresh air, it's not so fresh anymore.

If I wasn't concerned about other people's feelings, I would be wearing a mask all day every day. I keep a mask with me just in case I am in a place where I may get queasy. Not to mention wearing a glove. A lot of people do not clean or sanitize their hands. They wipe or pick their nose, they lick their fingers, scratch their head and other places.

Overall, invaders are invaders no matter how or where they come from. You must avoid them as much as possible. You will find that some doctors say invaders are good for you and they help build up your immune system. That may very well be true but for us, (people with lupus) it is not good. That is a death sentence.

As I speak of invaders, when I eat is when the real praying begins. When I consume various food items, I tend to have bacteria in my system for days. This means that the food could be undercooked, leftover from the night before, or contains bacteria from unclean hands. As a result, my gut is disturbed because of what I ingested, and now my immune system is contaminated with invaders. No healthy gut, no healthy body!

- When going out to eat buy a bottled drink or use a straw.
- If you are at a place getting a drink, I recommend that you do not get lemons added.
- Make sure the table, chairs, and eating utensils are clean.
- Do not use the cloth that is wrapped around your utensils to wipe your mouth. Ask for paper napkins.
- If the place smells LEAVE! The odor alone is an invader.

Most people know what bacteria are, but for those who do not, let me tell you. If you have any autoimmune system problems, microorganisms are not your friend. You will find that there are four types of bacteria, one of which is commonly found in your home or place of business.

For your home, indoor air has micrococcus, staphylococcus, bacillus, and pseudomonas. Bacteria is floating around everywhere and sitting on every surface, just waiting to jump up and infiltrate you. I have a purifier in my home to help pull some of the impurities out of the air. I find the purifier to be helpful.

Before I explain the different bacterias that are detrimental to our lives, I want to go back and explain more about the lemon. I know most of you were thinking "what", no! lemons. Lemons can perk up your drink by adding flavor, can benefit your health or just be a garnish. Depending on whether they wear gloves or wash their hands carefully, restaurant employees can spread bacteria when they are preparing the lemon slices. Unfortunately, several studies have found a significant number of bacteria (microbial growth) on lemon slices that can cause illness and disease. It can be difficult to know if the restaurant and bar employees handle lemons in an unsanitary way. Therefore, think twice before you order a lemon.

I want to provide you a visual of some of the invaders we must deal with:

Let's start with micrococcus, micrococcus is a sphere-shaped and relatively harmless bacterium. It is common on the skin, and can also be found in soil, water, dust and meat products. Micrococcus feeds on dead and decomposing materials and can cause spoilage of things like fish. This organism grows with oxygen and can also be responsible for causing an odor in human sweat. Micrococci have occasionally been reported as the cause of pneumonia, meningitis, and septic arthritis. Wear gloves when dealing with dirt. Drink water out of a closed container. Clean your meat with gloves on and keep your house or apartment clean from dust.

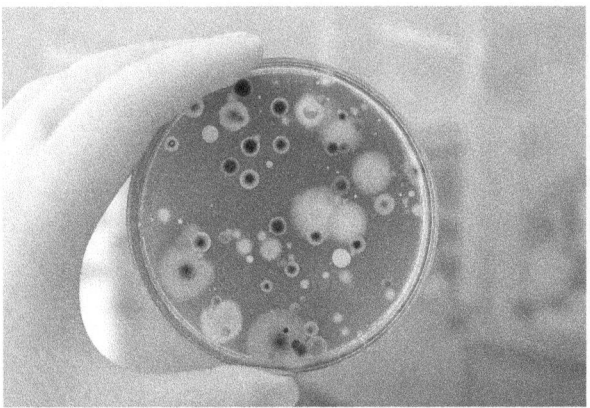

STAPHYLOCOCCUS

Staphylococcus is also a sphere-shaped bacterium and is well-known in hospitals. Staphylococcus is found virtually everywhere and may result in infection. This can be found in your throat, nasal passages and most of the time, these bacteria cause minor skin infections. Some medical professionals state that food poisoning and toxic shock syndrome are among the illnesses caused by staphylococcus. Not to mention, staphylococcus can grow with and without oxygen. So, work on getting a purifier for work and where you live.

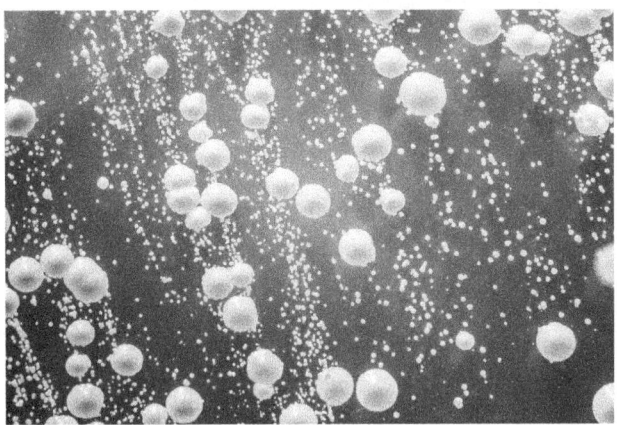

BACILLUS

Bacillus is a rod-shaped bacterium. It can be found within your digestive system. Some type of bacillus can cause food poisoning, illness, and infections. These toxins can cause two types of illness: one type characterized by diarrhea and the other, called an emetic toxin, by nausea and vomiting. These bacteria are present in foods and can multiply quickly at room temperature.

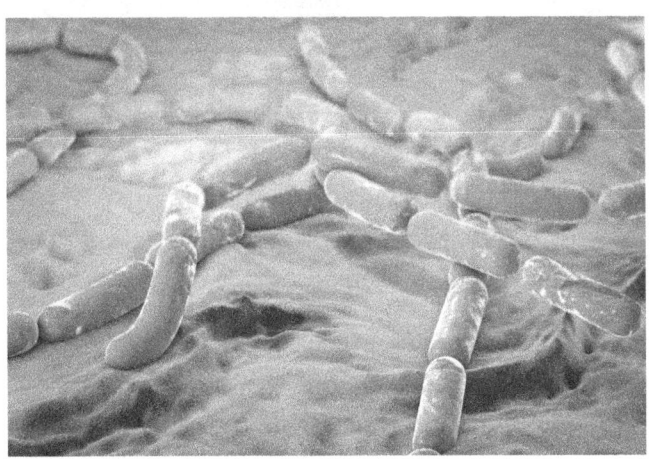

PSEUDOMONAS

Pseudomonas is another rod-shaped bacterium. This virus tends to only attack individuals who are immunocompromised (persons with weakened immune systems). The bacteria can be spread in hospitals via the hands of healthcare workers, or by hospital equipment that is not properly cleaned. Overall, the reason why it is important to understand the four (micrococcus, staphylococcus, bacillus, and pseudomonas) bacteria are usually one-celled microscopic living organisms, that can be found everywhere and can be dangerous to those with an autoimmune disease.

If you are a wine drinker STOP! The process of fermentation is wine decomposition which carries lots of bacteria. I am not sure if most people know about this but one thing you should know is that exposure to staphylococcus could lead to lupus. All sports arenas, playgrounds, locker rooms, bathrooms, and schools are playing fields for bacteria. The smallest amount of staphylococcus bacteria, which is frequently found on the skin or in the nose, could present a risk factor for developing chronic, inflammatory lupus. Other infections include those of the respiratory tract and urinary system.

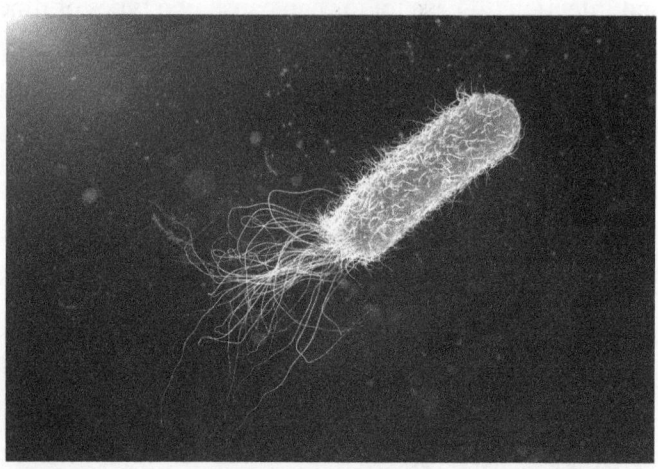

URINARY SYSTEM

The urinary tract includes the kidneys, ureters, bladder and the urethra. The purpose of urinary system is to eliminate waste from the body, regulate blood capacity, blood pressure, good levels of electrolytes, and metabolites. Inflammation within the kidneys that filter the blood, is called nephritis. Lupus nephritis is the word used when lupus causes inflammation in your kidneys, making them unable to accurately remove waste from your blood or control the number of fluids in your body. Abnormal numbers of waste can build up in the blood and swelling can acquire. If left untreated, nephritis can lead to long-lasting harm to the kidneys; causing you to need a kidney transplant.

In the early stages of lupus nephritis, there are very few signs that anything is wrong. Often the first indications of lupus nephritis are weight gain and puffiness in your feet, ankles, legs, and hands. It's predicted that up to 60 percent of all people with lupus, and as many as two-thirds of all children with lupus, will obtain kidney problems that need medical treatment. Testing your urine is very vital because there are so few indications of kidney disease. Significant harm to your kidneys can occur before you are diagnosed with lupus. Nephrologists are the doctors who treat and test to diagnose lupus nephritis.

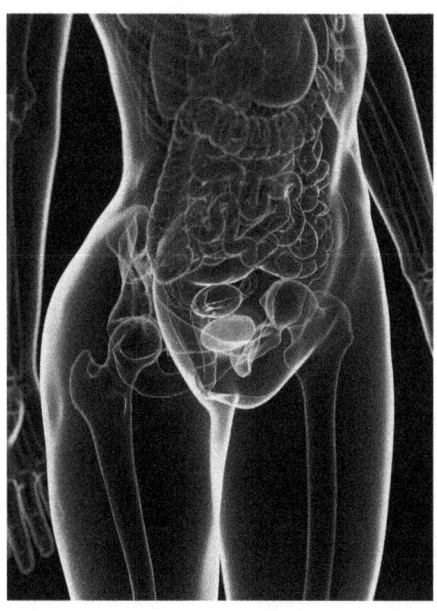

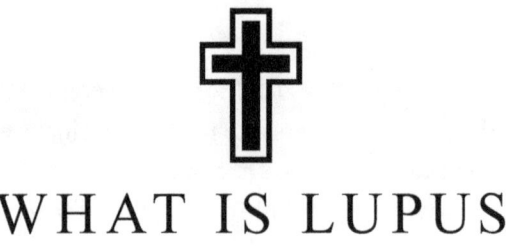

WHAT IS LUPUS

IT WAS IMPORTANT for me to explain about the invaders first before defining what lupus is. I wanted you to understand how germs affect your body. When defining lupus, you will have the invaders in the back of your mind, painting, a clear picture as you read about lupus. If you research on any website, for an example, WebMD (www.webmd.com/lupus), you will find that "Lupus is an autoimmune disease, where the immune system mistakes the body's tissues as an alien (which I call invaders) and attacks them." However, some people with lupus suffer only minor difficulties. While many who pass away have a death certificate that reads "unknown cause of death". Others must deal with a lifetime of unexplained disabilities.

God has a plan for you. Lupus affects more African Americans, less Asian, very few Native Americans and two to three times less Caucasians. Nine out of ten people with lupus are women. This disease usually strikes between birth and forty-four years of age. It can occur in older people as well because of late diagnosis. This could also be because it was overlooked at a younger age, which happened to me.

There are many types of lupus but only two I will discuss:

- The discoid lupus erythematosus (DLE)
- The systemic lupus erythematosus (SLE).

DLE is located where the skin is exposed to sunlight. It produces skin lacerations that often leave marks after the healing of the wounds. DLE can sometimes be mistaken for vitiligo. Vitiligo is a disease in which the pigment is lost from parts of the skin, causing white or pale patches, often with no reason. It doesn't usually affect essential organs.

I was tested by a dermatologist, who later referred me to an outside specialist. After two years, the specialist still could not understand why I had light patches on my face, arms, and back. At one point in time, I was placed in a tube with ultraviolet lights for minutes, four days out of the week. This treatment was to see if the pale patches would go away or darken. After three years of wasted time and money with no change, it was time to give up. I will explain more about this later as I continue the talk about lupus and celebrities it has affected.

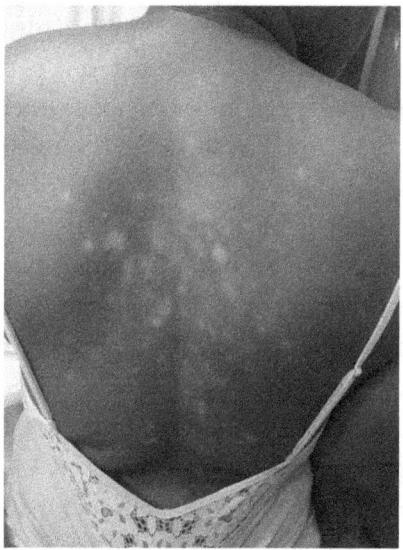

Vitiligo is a disease that causes the loss of skin color in blotches. The extent of color loss from vitiligo are unpredictable. It affects the skin on any part of your body. It may also affect the hair and the inside of the mouth.

Michael Jackson (1958–2009) was an American singer, songwriter, actor, and dancer who, per the media, had vitiligo. Many wondered if that was the reason his skin color altered severely as he got older. Stress can worsen your condition, but it can be treated by applying topical steroids and using ultraviolet lights. However, with lupus (SLE), you must stay away from ultraviolet light and sunlight. As for me, having SLE ultraviolet light caused many migraine headaches.

As I continued my research, I was surprised to find a few more people, like NBA player Rasheed Wallace, NFL player J.D. Runnels, Singers Tamar Braxton, and Rigo Tovar (1946–2005), they've all dealt with a form of an immune system issue. The main reason for the loss of pigmentation is due to dysfunctional autoimmune systems that destroys the skin color, but no one knows why. I think this is one thing that needs to be researched and yes, on humans.

I found a way to take care of my skin by keeping the skin clean with all-natural products or dermatology recommended soaps. Drink lots of water (purified drinking water, not mineral, spring or distilled because it could have a counter effect with supplements/medication), and take vitamins (A, C, D, and E) to produce and maintain a well immune system. I found that when the season changes, the pigmentation of my skin changes its appearance.

SLE is more serious. It affects the skin and other vital organs. SLE can cause flat butterfly rash across the bridge of the nose and cheeks. It can also affect other parts of the skin elsewhere on the body, like your back, ears, chest, and arms. Aside from the visible effects of SLE, the illness may also inflame and/or damage the connective tissue in the joints, muscles, the membranes nearby the skin, lungs, heart, kidneys and the brain. However, one of my doctors said that brain involvement is rare.

As for me, it was different. When going to visit my neurologist, I was told that I had two inches of intracranial air in my brain that the doctor wanted to remove to stop the pressure that causes my headaches. That was a "no", as my husband refused the procedure. The air is called Pneumocephalus. Pneumocephalus is the presence of air within the cranial cavity. My CT scans for tension pneumocephalus showed air that compresses the frontal lobes of my brain, which results in a tented appearance of the brain in the skull known as the Mount Fuji sign.

I know you want to know what happens when the Pneumocephalus compresses the frontal lobe of the brain. Well, when an air bubble enters a vein, it's called a venous air embolism. When an air bubble enters an artery, it's called an arterial air embolism. These air bubbles can travel to your brain, heart, or lungs and cause a heart attack, stroke, or respiratory failure. It can be treated by having skull-base surgery. One would manage with conservative measures such as bed rest, head elevation, supplemental oxygen via a face tent or 100% nonrebreather with absolute avoidance of positive pressure, and pain control.

When speaking with my neurologist to find out what causes pneumocephalus. He explained that the majority of pneumocephalus cases are due to trauma. I have had lots of trauma over the years. At one point, I was hit upside the head with a piggy bank. I was in a bad relationship and was beat and left for dead. Overall, stress is the new killer, and more will be discussed later in the book.

Lupus for me causes confusion, depression, flogs, seizures, and even strokes, which happened to me in my twenties. I have every symptom that SLE has to offer. I am not pleased about it by any means, but I do know that God has a plan. I have seen so many doctors, and not one of them can tell me what causes lupus. If you want to know if anyone is working on a cure, the answer is yes. Researchers are working to find the cause of lupus, but as of now, there is no true answer to a cure.

I decided to take matters into my own hands and monitor my body for ten years to see what was going on with me. By the age of twenty-five, I had Graves' disease, intestinal problems, and heart problems. By thirty, it was lupus. I am knocking on fifty's door, and guess what? It is still lupus but in remission or as described by some doctors in the family of "arthritis".

For the past 30 years, I have seen an extraordinary increase in consumer demand for safe, effective, and cost-effective natural health care plans. So, I decided to reach out to see a Naturopathic doctor.

Naturopathic supplements have emerged in the health-care profession as being best suited to meet the demand of people's needs. Although it almost disappeared in the mid-twentieth century because of the popularity of drugs and surgery, naturopathic supplements now offers safe, effective natural therapies as a vital part of the new health-care systems of North America in the twenty-first century. Naturopathic physicians are trained in the art and science of natural health care at accredited medical colleges. Integrative partnerships between conventional medical doctors and licensed NDs are becoming more available. It also increases patient satisfaction in their relationships with their care providers. More people are adding naturopathic supplements to their health-care options. When doing my research, it cost between $200 to $500 per visit. I was flabbergasted. Saddened, over time, I was not able to continue my treatments due to a shortage of funds. However, I received great information, when the time comes, and I have money to visit a naturopathic physician I will continue using their services.

> *A woman is not defeated when losing; A woman is defeated when A woman quits. Do not quit. Make that change in your life.*
>
> —LaTonya Bias, PhD

Note: Motivation

> *Believe in your heart that you are healed. The disease is a body that is not at ease; man or woman becomes what he or she thinks about.*
>
> —LaTonya Bias, PhD

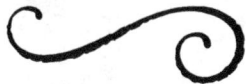

WHAT CAUSES LUPUS?

YOU NEED TO understand and pay close attention to your body. No solitary factor is known to cause lupus. Research suggests that a mixture of hereditary (Genetics), hormonal (Cytokines), environmental, and immune system factors may be behind it all. I would agree. Environmental issues alter from virus-related bacterial infections to severe emotional stress. Overexposure to cold and hot weather implies that it is also a role in lupus.

The normal, healthy immune system protects against intruders, such as viruses, bacteria, or toxins by increasing what is called an immune response. This response comes in two key approaches: immune cells and protein antibodies. There are two core types of immune cells.

T cells, which are the suppressor cells, and B cells, which push the cells to produce the antibodies. In lupus, there is a reduced suppressor response called invaders, and the worker B cells go into overdrive and create extra antibodies. These antibodies can in turn cause damage to vital body parts, such as the blood vessels and the blood cells.

It has been said that certain drugs, such as blood pressure drugs, may cause lupus and can go undetected by a specialist. In simple terms, lupus is thought to be a condition with a traditional tendency for the immune system to go into overdrive.

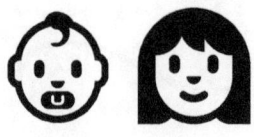

WHY IS GENETICS IMPORTANT TO LUPUS?

GENETICS ARE IMPORTANT to understand because one would wonder how one developed lupus. There are days when I am thinking back on how and when this could have happened. Why me, why me? I just found myself researching, looking for answers daily. I was reaching and reaching for any answer I could get from blogs, people, and Lupus Foundations. I joined a foundation to see what information I could get that would help provide answers. Let me just say that my questions still went unanswered.

I investigated a study by Hughes, G. (2009), which explained a twin study from the London Lupus Centre. They have shown believably that lupus has a hereditary tendency. Lupus patients often have family histories of lupus or other autoimmune diseases. The most common types are rheumatoid arthritis, multiple sclerosis, and Sjogren's syndrome. The study of twins was interesting because the chance of an identical twin developing the illness is 60 percent. For the geneticist, this would propose two things; one, lupus has a deep genetic tendency, two, this genetic predisposition not only factored in the disease but also the environment.

My genetic makeup is predominantly shown to be my father's side. My grandmother had twins; one had a disability (RIP). One would think that whatever my uncle had it was passed down to me. My grandmother and aunt on my father's side passed away from cancer may they RIP. This sparked me to investigate if one could find any affiliation between cancer and lupus.

In 2009, mice were used by researchers to find any missing links related to cancer. Research has been done for a long time. They have been so busy fighting to find a cure for Cancer and AIDS that the severity of lupus has not been addressed and is growing by the minute. Lots of money has been generated for these causes and someday we may have a cure. However, this is not acceptable because lupus should be treated with the same level of importance as Cancer and AIDS. This will be explained in part 2 of the Lupus journey.

I plan to speak and write until the world knows about the depths of lupus and that there is a cure. You can help me. Tell people to read this book or simply gift this book to someone you know. Wear purple in May and donate to lovelifelupusfoundation.org, for the cause. This would be of much help to the people with invaders in their bodies and research for a cure.

Dwight H. Kono and Argyrios N. Theofilopouuos (2009), from Genetics of Systemic Autoimmunity in Mouse Models of Lupus: International evaluations of immunology explains that systemic lupus erythematosus (SLE) is genetic as a multifaceted polygenic trait, connecting genetic, environmental, and stochastic issues. I did not know what stochastic was, so it was time to find out. I found that "Stochastic is when having an unintentional change, a pattern may be inspected statistically but may not remain predicted accurately." That is interesting. The researcher states that in these beginning developments, it has been difficult to find progress that has been made toward the clarification of the hereditary basis for stochastic. In addition to this approach, transgenic studies have launched to classify genetic factors that can stimulate autoimmunity in non-autoimmune and lupus-prone background in mice. Think about that for a minute. Anyway!

The inconsistencies this theory has is all based on mice, one would never find the same results in a human. How do I know? Because I was one of those mice. I don't find that inspiring at all, but this is the type of research that I would come across. When I found out about my illness, I was sick because I would classify myself in the same study as the mice. As I research more, I find that most scientists in the United States will not provide their research on lupus. It's not an open book. People are afraid to speak out, and I would like to know if mice or humans play a major factor in their results. All you hear is millions of people have been diagnosed and people talk about family members or friends passing away for unknown reasons. As my search continued, I wanted to know where this illness generated, if other countries hand anything to do with it, or if they have a cure.

A China study was done by L. Mu, 2018, discovering the humanity and causes of death in Chinese patients with systemic lupus erythematosus. It was great to know that Mr. Mu collected the clinical data of all successful adult systemic lupus erythematosus patients at the rheumatology division of Peking University First Hospital between January 2007 and December 2015. I called Peking University to see if additional notes from the study were open for the public to view. I was advised it was not for the public. Besides I was given the run around, so as I read the information Mr. Mu had in his article. Mr. Mu explained that the main causes of death acknowledged the consistent humanity ratio and years of life lost were calculated. The variables (lifestyle, the food they eat) associated with humanity were determined by Kaplan-Meier's and Cox's regression analysis separately. I could go on, but the conclusion stated the humankind of systemic lupus erythematosus patients in China was considerable in females, associated with toxicity as the leading cause of death. Old age infection, autoimmune hemolytic anemia, thrombocytopenia, and pulmonary arterial hypertension were met with unfortunate results. Wow, so what this study was telling me, I need to watch what I ate and how I worked out. Even if you are paying attention to your body, consult a naturopathic doctor and have your Th1 and Th2 checked out. The first thing a naturopathic doctor will do is clean your gut from the toxicity. Gut dysfunctions appear to be causing wrong bacteria to formulate in your gut. Resulting in unhealthy metabolites (toxins) entering body. You will be surprised how it all relates to your illness. That was a lot of big words. I still find it hard to pronounce them all. Erythema… what, Stochastic… who?

However, as we continue, there are days when I don't feel good and it could just be the cytokines interacting between my body cells. Cytokines are small secreted proteins released by cells that have a specific effect on the interactions and communications between your cells. Cytokines' hormonal messengers are responsible for most of the biological effects in your immune system, such as cells' mediate immunity and allergic-type responses.

Although they are numerous, cytokines can be functionally divided into two groups: those that are pro-inflammatory (causing inflammation) and those that are essentially anti-inflammatory (reduce inflammation) but promote allergic responses. You would need to pay attention to your body. Listen closely, because for me, inflammation happens during the day, and I would have to take supplements (not medication) to reduce the swelling. Recommendation: check with your Ear, Nose, and Throat Specialist (ENT) to have a full allergy test done. This way, you will know what you are allergic too and you can take control of your life.

You hear people say, "my bones hurt" or "the weather is about to change I feel it". Well, it's true when you have Lupus. Your five senses (touch, sight, hearing, smell and taste) are unique so the information sent to your brain will help you understand what is going on with your body so listen. T lymphocytes are a major source of cytokines. T cells or T lymphocytes are a type of white blood cell that plays a role in developing stem cells in your bone marrow and circulate the body scanning for cellular abnormalities. They help protect the body from infection or our invaders. They can also recognize normal tissue during episodes or what I call flare-ups of your autoimmune system.

The gaps are the devastating effects of when a lower-than-normal number of just one type of T-cells are obvious. This could show that you don't have any problems when your test results come back making them killer cell after cells that are infected by a virus. Now you could be misdiagnosed and provided something to treat just an infection for whatever invader the doctor sees stand out the most. This would be a case when you go to the doctor to get tested for lupus and they state you do not have the autoimmune disease.

One very important note to remember; knowing the difference between your molecules allows you to know what to look for when you are having your yearly blood exam. Have a full blood panel done. Most doctors do not do it because your insurance will not cover it. It is also good to know what is responsible for killing intracellular parasites and for perpetuating the autoimmune responses. Read more about that in part 2 of the next book *Does CBD & MARIJUANA Help Lupus?*

You may think, *"Oh, I will just detox and I will be fine."* Well, there is more to that. Th1-type cytokine's important responsibility is to produce proinflammatory responses. Too many proinflammatory responses can lead to uncontrolled tissue damage, so there needs to be something put in place to counteract this. Today, I work with a naturopathic doctor that provides supplements to help balance my system.

When talking about balancing my system. My challenges are *sugar* and *salt*. I cannot have one without the other. Since I have a challenged immune system, there is no way I will produce the right balance. Sometimes when I crave a lot of sweets or sugary drinks (pop or soda), it's parasites in me driving my desires. I told my doctor one day that I think I have parasites in my body. He asked me a lot of questions and determined that I did not have parasites. No testing was done. When I went to see a naturopathic doctor, I was advised that more 60 million Americans are walking about with different type of parasites one called toxoplasmosis.

Parasites vary depending on what region you live in. However, I was advised that one way to slow down but not kill off the parasites, is to stop eating sugar. This is what is keeping them alive.

The only time I would stop the intake of sugar and salt is when I wanted to dramatically lose weight. Just that loss of sugar and salt not only helped with slowing down the life of parasites but drinking lots of water will help to get their eggs and dead bodies flushed out of my system. In part 2 of the next book called *Does CBD & MARIJUANA Help Lupus*. I will go into more detail. Today, the world has everyone thinking that different types of sugar is better to use. What I have learned is "sugar is sugar".

We have parents, Millennials and Gen Z, moving towards having the right to decide if they want their child(ren) to get vaccinated. It is all about a parent's rights. Could having shots for example, the flu be a part of how autoimmune disease are being created? Diversity of genes can independently or in combination promote systemic autoimmunity in mice. This complexity, which is also observed in human with lupus, emphasizes the importance of using experimental and less-complex mouse models to define these processes, a tactic that has already generated new insights. I hope this helps you with your illness. Remember to continue to follow the light and God will guide your footsteps.

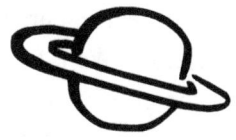

ENVIRONMENT

SOME PEOPLE SAY they had a bad upbringing, but I want to say that I didn't. Was I poor? Yes. Did I live in bad locations and environments? Yes. I had family who loved me unconditionally, and God ordering my steps. However, the choices I made in life were not so great. I remember playing in nasty parks, abandoned buildings, and vacant lots. When I was able to work, I cleaned vacant apartments, worked in nasty kitchens, and lived in unsafe environments. Could that have been a contributing factor? It is possible!

Not sure about back in the 1970s but today your environment outside of your home is very important. Why? Maintaining a healthy environment is essential to increasing the quality of life. Globally, 23% of all deaths and 26% of deaths among children under age five, are due to preventable environmental factors. Your environment can influence your behavior and motivate changes in your mood. For example, the results of several research studies reveal that rooms with bright lights, both natural and artificial, can improve health outcomes such as depression, agitation, and even sleep. Also, environmental factors trigger my lupus and offset my progressions such as smells, dirt, dust, perfumes, and ultraviolet light.

Growing up on the south side of Chicago, many landlords did not take good care of their properties. I think that uninhabitable living conditions caused some of my health issues. I can remember a time when living in low-income apartments on the inside the apartment stayed clean. However, on the outside of the apartments, the city did not keep up grass, trash or remove any stray cats or dogs. You had to be very careful going upstairs because you could fall through them. I could never understand why we had so many roaches. No matter how much you clean they continued to multiply, leaving behind shells from reproducing more babies. Could cleaning up dead roaches be a factor in me having an autoimmune disease? Well, let me research roaches. Lol! When researching if roaches can give you a disease, I found that roaches eat a wide range of food, including rotten garbage. I had to clean lots of feces, dead roaches, and rats. I cleaned without a mask with germs floating around that could harm your body. The things that our family ate, and our living environment, could also have played a major part in why I have a disability. It is believed that they spread several diseases to humans including salmonella and gastroenteritis. Recent studies have indicated roaches can also cause allergies. What are the odds of that? It could be the roaches taking me out; save me, Lord. Lol!

Do tell..., most was talked about at the beginning of this book. However, I lived in low-income housing (environmental). I attended a school that had a lack of funding, and my world felt like it was every man for themselves. As a child, I went to church with my father's mother and participated in the choir, but by the time I went into high school, I hate to say this, but I put my best friend (God) to the side because I lost my grandmother. My grandmother was a dedicated woman. She was God-fearing and loved her family. She kept me grounded in Christ. The streets became my best friend. I was lost until I became an adult at the age of eighteen. I can remember having health problems when I was young, but I did not understand why. I went to the bathroom once a month, if that, to have a bowel movement and urinated once a day. I could not go to the bathroom outside my home. Still to this day, I have an ongoing issue. Never did I think to speak up or ask someone in my family if they have the same health issue. I thought it was normal.

I would always have heavy periods that would go for two to three weeks and lots of headaches. I never wanted to go anywhere because I was tired all the time. However, the family stepped in with lots of encouragement, and I was able to get back on my feet within a year. "Every little step I take," they would be there. "Every little step I made," we would be together. Go Bobby, Brown!

You know what? There is something about God's love that just knocks you off your feet. I found that I was one of those people who would call on God when I needed him, and God would show up right on time. He never left me because I went through some tough times in my life. He has always let me know that I am his child of God.

One day I had a long day at work. I was very tired and weak and wanted to just lay down, but when I came home, there were other things to do around the house, with family, the dog, etc. It was late when I went to bed, but I was not that sleepy. As I was resting, my tongue started to itch, then came a sharp pain. Now what? I got up, went into the bathroom, and looked at my tongue in the mirror. I thought, *Okay, I think we have another situation.* I could not close my mouth, or I would not be able to breathe. You know that the tongue is a muscular organ in the mouth and is used in the act of swallowing. I was not sure why, but I was having a hard time breathing. I was thinking about what I could have eaten that would cause my tongue to grow the size of a lemon. I waited and waited, thinking it was just me, and allowed hours to go by. However, it got to the point, I could feel my tongue getting bigger and bigger in my mouth. At the time my family only had one car, and my husband was gone to work. I did not know what to do. I could not talk, so I could not call 911. Thank God there was an emergency room down the street.

I walked to the emergency room and found out that I was having a mild stroke. I advised the doctors at three o'clock in the morning that I had lupus, and they looked as if they did not know what to do. I was left in the room for hours after taking the medication that they gave to take the swelling down. The doctors came back and asked what the hospital would give me if I was having a flare-up. I explained the cocktail, but they did not get it. The doctors came back and told me to follow up with my primary doctor. They told me the swelling should go down in a few hours, and if not, I should return to the emergency room. They told me, I was having a mini-stroke and asked how I got to the hospital. I advised that I walked, the doctors looked at each other and one of them said, "we are going to send you home, why did you walk?" I explained.

I understood and called my rheumatologist the next day. She gave me a prescription for an EpiPen. The rheumatologist advised that I needed to keep the EpiPen on me always. After they ran blood work and lots of tests, it was found to be a stroke, but no one could tell me how it happened and what to do if it happens again. Enough is enough. I could not complete my goals in life or take the next steps to move forward because I kept having issues. Why? I don't know, and no doctor knows.

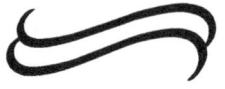

FAMILY

IT IS GOOD to have family members who can somehow make you understand their logic in life. My family members would always say, "Life is about the choices you make." As for me, it took years, well until I turned twenty-something, for me to understand. I was making a lot of bad choices. You undergo a lifetime of disappointments, by listening to your friends, having the wrong role model, or even second-guessing yourself. When I was younger, I would think that my life was an action-packed movie, for example, everywhere I turned it was always something. You can be in your feelings or think your "life is like a box of chocolates and you never know what you are going to get" (Forest Gump). However, I found over the years that the best answer for that is to seek God to guide your path.

> The Lord is my shepherd; I shall not want. He makes me lie down in green pastures, he leads me beside still waters, he restores my soul, he leads me in paths of righteousness for his name's sake. Even though I walk through the valley of the shadow of death, I will fear no evil, for you are with me; your rod and your staff, they comfort me. You prepare a table before me in the presence of my enemies. You anoint my head with oil, my cup overflows. Surely goodness and love will follow me all the days of my life, and I will dwell in the house of the Lord forever. (Psalm 23:1–6 ESV)

My family members, well, first, I know you are wondering, "Why is this writer saying, 'my family members, my family members'?" To clear this up, I must keep the family names out of this book. If I say one name in my family, all the rain that turns hard is going to break loose. So, I will use pseudonyms as descriptors.

I can hear my family members or friends saying, "What kind of sugar, honey, ice, tea (put the first letter of every word together to understand what I am saying) is this? Are you telling the world about me? What is wrong with you? You are becoming weak? (punk) What are you thinking? You have lost your mind? You think you are better than us?" Understanding that a lot of people, my family in general, from Chicago do not talk about their business. The truth is people need to know and understand what is wrong with you so that your health will not affect generations to come.

Sorry! you will find I will ramble a lot or go down rabbit trails throughout the book about my family and friends to ease some of the seriousness of this topic. No way am I denying the significance of lupus because I have lupus. Lupus is my journey but not my life, that is why I want to provide insight into my experience(s). I know you are ready to dive into the heart of lupus. However, give me a few pages of your time and I will lay it out for you.

Back to what family would say. My family member would also say, "You are what you eat." When adults tell you things like that, you'd better believe them. As for me, I found that hard to believe back in the day, but boy, I should have listened. When I was young and smelling myself, I would always listen to my friends and go back and tell my family, "You don't know what you are talking about." My family would hate that expression but would say, "You will learn." How I wish I would have listened. However, my family would never say things that would make me feel bad.

My family was always telling me things that made me think about life. Did I listen? No, no, no. This relates to my lupus because if I would have listened and eaten right when I was younger or made the right choices in life, my path in life would be a bit different.

Word of advice: Listen up and pay attention; when you are around family members such as your parents or elders, please ask questions about their medical background, you must know. Don't wait until you are sick to ask. Not knowing could be crucial but knowing is key. Do you know your blood type? Find out now. Never did anyone in my family tell me about sickness, diseases, or things in my upbringing that could have led me to have so many health issues. I did not think to ask because very few people were sick in my family. If they were, my family was very good at keeping it from me. I would hear, "Aunt Boo died" or "Your cousin CC died," not knowing how or why. Never did I ask. Take the importance of this message and note that you need to talk with your family. Ask questions and if you get cursed out don't get mad, explain why. If you cannot get an answer do some research.

> There is a time for everything, and a season for every activity under heaven: a time to be born and a time to die. (Ecclesiastes 3:2 ESV)

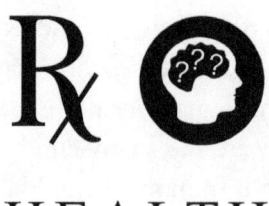

HEALTH

And who had suffered much under many physicians, and had spent all that she/he had, and was no better but rather grew worse. (Mark 5:26 ESV)

I CAN REMEMBER having lower stomach pain and could not explain why. People would ask all the time "are you alright?" I would tell them, yes, but I wanted to say no. The only reason I would say yes only to avoid the hospital. At this point in my life, I did not feel like doing anything but staying in bed. I have missed out on so much during that time that as of today I have placed all my tasks on my bucket list. The pain became excruciating over the years, to the point when a sharp pain would hit me, I was bent over. I could not sit for a long time. For example, in elementary school, my attention span was very short because I was in pain but did not know how to explain it. I could remember being very creative, writing short story books, being a hairdresser on my dolls, knitting, and counting the cars out of the window every night when I went to bed until I could go to sleep, hoping the pain would go away. Never did I connect the pain with something I ate or my environment.

After seeing many doctors for bacteria issues that were causing pain in several areas in my body, I could not believe this was happening to me. Do you know what lupus is? Most people don't. You find people saying it's like HIV and look at you funny or saying it's an infection in your blood. No, nowhere near correct. What does lupus look like? Does anyone know? There is no look other than for some people like me you have white spots on your face or your body. The lupus diagnosis is increasing day by day. There is a lack of awareness in people, companies, doctor-errs, yes, I said it, doctors-errs, family, and your friends. They do not understand what lupus is about. If you looked at me, you would not know I have lupus because I look like nothing is wrong with me. Lupus does not have a face or expressions that will tell someone, "Oh she has lupus." People with lupus smile, sing, dance, crack jokes, walk, talk, make love, make mistakes and bleed like everyone else. The only difference is we have flare-ups. Please note that for more severe cases, these actions do not take place. When a flare-up occurs, 90 percent of my time is spent in bed the other 10 percent is work. No one wants to live that way. However, when you have lupus, you must make the best of it.

My health is so bad that my goal is to explain to the world what I know from my personal experience with lupus. After you read this book, you will learn what a day is like when one has an autoimmune disease. Not only that, I wrote this book so it could inform people who just don't understand. For example, my job placed me on desk duty because they did not want me to hurt anyone when they found out I had lupus. That told me, they did not understand what Lupus is about. My friends wonder why I cannot remember their birthdays, and why I do not call or hang out that much. The world looks at you funny when they see you have all those funny-looking white spots on your face, arms, and back. I was ashamed when the spots appeared on my face. I could not go anywhere without trying to cover up the white spots. I did not know it was on my back until I saw it on my chest, and I asked my husband to check. Some people are limited in the clothes they wear because of the spots on their bodies. I am sorry, I am getting very emotional right now because it is very stressful trying to explain what lupus is about. "BUT I HAVE TO GET THE WORD OUT". Sorry! Those who have lupus know that stress is deadly. Before I go further, let me explain stress and acknowledge a few people.

WHAT IS STRESS

Therefore, I tell you, do not worry about your life, what you will eat or drink; or about your body, what you will wear. Is not life more important than food, and the body more important than clothes? (Matthew 6:25 ESV)

STRESS IS DEFINED as an organism's whole reaction to environmental pressures. When stress was first considered in the 1950s, the term represents both the causes and the knowledgeable effects of these stresses. Today the word *stressor* has been used for the stimulus that provokes a stress response. Stress in humans results from interactions between persons, an environment that is perceived as straining or exceeding their capacities and threatening their well-being. Stress responses reflect differences in personality, as well as differences in physical strength or general health as illustrated below.

Stress Curve

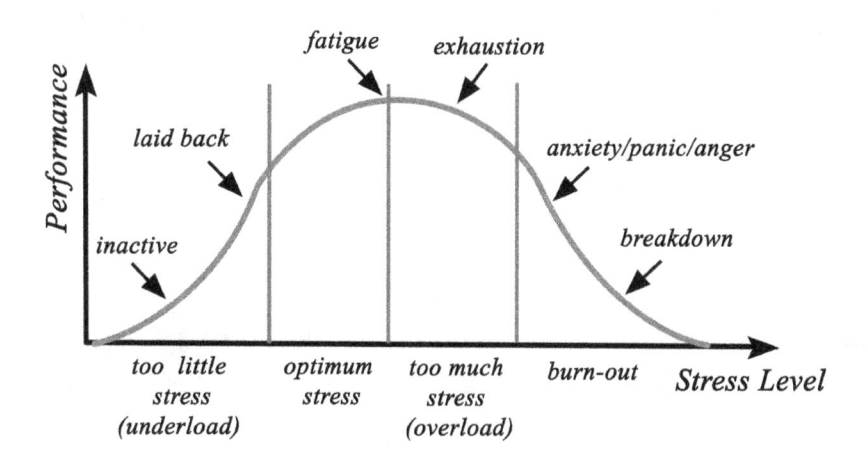

Performance (y-axis) vs *Stress Level* (x-axis)

- inactive
- laid back
- fatigue
- exhaustion
- anxiety/panic/anger
- breakdown

x-axis labels: too little stress (underload) — optimum stress — too much stress (overload) — burn-out

As illustrated above, stress results in increased productivity up to a point, after which things go rapidly downhill in your life. Beside that point or peak differs for each of us, so you need to be sensitive to the early warning symptoms telling you that you are overloaded starting to push you over the hump. Not to mention, many times, we create our stress because of flawed perceptions we can learn to correct. I want to tell you to move from the back of the bus to the front, and as Eleanor Roosevelt noted, "Nobody can make you feel inferior without your consent." While everyone can't agree on a definition of stress, clinical research confirms that the sense of having little or no control is always distressful.

Let me explain on how to be a stress-free person when dealing with Lupus or with someone you know that has Lupus. You have a responsibility before God to consistently get better, and one of the most reliable ways to do that is to be true to yourself. Here are a few steps that I do: Never make promises to yourself that you cannot keep. For example, I am going to work out today and you don't go. You tell yourself I will do it tomorrow. You are not guaranteed tomorrow, so do it when you plan it do not put it off. It's ok to make a mistake. Slipups are not made to make people feel better. When oversights are made it help you work to ease your mind of stress after you know what to do to correct the wrong you have done.

Next, being mad at the world. Keep a smile on your face, greet people, and make the most out of every day. This will help improve your day each time you focus on loving life. The problems are not within you but within the people who don't understand you. Life always judging the book by the cover. Continue to show that your cover is happy no matter how you feel.

Last, you tell yourself; I got help! I don't need anyone. You can get help with stress. When you are going to the doctor, some things they recommend avoiding when having a migraine or dealing with stress are to stay away from high-magnesium foods like Chinese food, onions, and some vinegar. Magnesium is good for you, which I will explain later. Other foods to avoid if you are dealing with stress are:

- peanut butter, nuts, pizza, avocadoes, anything fermented like sausage and wine, salami, pepperoni, baloney, hot dogs, pickled or marinated, chicken livers, sour cream, hot fresh bread, donuts, canned foods, chocolate, yogurt, lima and navy beans, peapods, tea, coffee, cola, excessive citrus foods, excessive pork, excessive bananas, and whipped and cheddar cheeses and any SUGARS. I know you are thinking, *Well, what I am going to eat?* I said the same thing, but fruit and vegetables and no meat will be your new friend.

To continue, you should avoid alcoholic beverages, especially champagne, beer, wines, gin, and vodka. Some doctors would say having a glass of wine a day will keep the doctor away. Well, not for us. It's interesting how the little things I love trigger migraine or stress. Work in stress-free environments, read, listen to music or do a light workout. These are the items I found helpful for me.

Oh, I almost forgot, find a doctor who can provide you with a skin allergy test. The reason for this is a part of getting to know your body. Your test results allow you to know what you are allergic too. A skin allergy test or prick test is a method for diagnosing allergies that attempts to provoke a small, controlled allergic response. If you have severe generalized skin disease or an acute skin infection, you should not undergo a skin test.

If you have DLE (discoid lupus erythematosus), your doctor might suggest a different type of testing. Always check with your doctor first but I would recommend a naturopathic doctor. Naturopathic supplements are a system that uses natural remedies to help the body heal itself. You can also do a blood test that will measure specific antibodies in the blood to determine if you have allergies. My test came back that I am allergic to everything. Knowing this information will help you pay attention to your body. You will know what to eat, what to sleep on, wear, or be around after having this test done. All your stress factor will reduce as you become knowledgeable about yourself. "Knowledge is Power!"

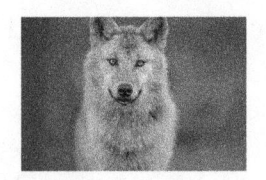

THE WOLF

THE WORD LUPUS can be called "the wolf" or appear as a butterfly (which is the lupus symbol) because many people with lupus-like myself develop a butterfly-shaped spot over their cheeks and nose that gives them something of a wolf-like an appearance. The spots may appear on other parts of the body, such as your chest, ears, hands, shoulders, upper arms, and even your back. There are three types of lupus that affect your skin Discoid Lupus Erythematosus (DLE), Subacute Cutaneous Lupus Erythematosus (SCLE), and Tumid Lupus). A skin biopsy is usually obtained to diagnose skin lupus, and each form possesses its characteristic lesions and pattern. However, according to the "Americans on the Top: American Rheumatologist Association," many symptoms must occur either seriously or at the same time before a diagnosis can be made.

The butterfly spots on your cheeks could mean that you have a low white blood cell count. That is why some rheumatologists will send you to see a dermatologist. A butterfly spot can be known as a malar rash and is described as a skin irritation that extends across the face in a butterfly appearance. A butterfly spot is one of the signs of Lupus Erythematosus. Butterfly spots are usually a symptom and not a condition. However, they still have no cure.

Butterfly spots (Malar) rashes are not serious, but they may be itchy and quite painful in some cases. Butterfly spots are like rashes that appear in type 1 diabetes, type 2 diabetes, and psoriasis. Butterfly flushing or spots may occur as a clinical feature of various immune-related conditions.

Although the exact cause is not known, people with rosacea appear red and flushed in the face due to blood-vessel enlargement. Acute renal failure may cause symptoms related to uremia and fluid overload. Acute nephritic disease may manifest as hypertension and hematuria.

Other disorders that can cause a butterfly rash to appear are worth mentioning, and one of the more common disorders is dermatomyositis. It is very important to understand about the butterfly spots when speaking with your dermatologist, he or she will not pull your leg for information. He or she will see that you understand your body. When you go for treatment, it depends on which organs are affected and how active the inflammation is taken place. Timely treatment can control and reduce the flare-up of lupus butterfly spots on your face. Do not let someone tell you that cream will do the job. It did not work for me, but it may work for you, but I have been through a lot of creams and different skin care treatments, and nothing works. However, you will notice that in the summer, your spots will become darker and in the colder months, they will become lighter. Therefore, I always stay covered.

As I explained, the most common way of diagnosis of malar rash is to undergo blood tests, urine tests, and biopsy of the kidneys. The diagnosis of lupus is generally made clinically, that is, based on the symptoms you are experiencing. When a diagnosis of lupus has not yet been made, one of the presenting symptoms that commonly assists diagnosis is the presence of a spot projecting on the face, arms, or back. You may have mouth sores, seizures, be sensitive to light, and your tongue could swell, as all this happen to me. A specific antibody that is found in people can be up to 50 percent lupus symptoms. Sometimes you might even have to get a kidney biopsy that may need to be diagnosed as lupus. Otherwise, you may get recommendations to see a rheumatologist. That means, you know you are going to the right place, understand that naturopathic doctor is better.

NATURAL PLANTS DAILY

NATURAL PLANT BASED things you can take to help you with your daily function are calcium (leafy dark greens like spinach, collard, and kale) and magnesium (bananas, kelp, and oats) that are essential for pH balance and protection against bone loss due to your arthritis. I would advise the best brand, but I don't want to support anyone and end up getting feedback. However, the recommended daily dose for calcium magnesium is 1500 mg daily. For calcium, take from 15 to 3,000 mg daily. The next nutritional supplement that is recommended is a vitamin C release of 2,000 mg daily. Kelp is also essential to recommend. If your tummy gets upset a lot, try to avoid milk, eggs or any dairy. I do recommend a good diet and no meat or seafood. Plant Base Only.

Eating a plant-base meal keeps your body from reacting negatively, allowing me to have less flare up and is easy on my kidneys. Use only plant-base oils. Considering you know good sources of essential fatty acids, if you feel as though you must eat, try to eat eggs, garlic, or onions and small portions of meat (protein). The best thing is to become a vegetarian. I try not to eat too many eggs. I love the rice but do not drink much milk. Having high blood pressure, rice must go. These foods contain sulfur, which is needed for the repair and rebuilding of the bones and connective tissues. I take vitamin D for that nutrition.

You can include in your diet with brown rice, fish, green, leafy vegetables, fresh fruit (sugar), and oatmeal that is whole grain.

Eat fresh pineapples frequently, not canned. The enzymes in fresh pineapples are an excellent source for reducing inflammation. As soon as I feel one sharp pain or weather change, I run to the pineapple. What about water? I found out that some waters are not good for me. As for me, I drink water that has enzymes. I do not drink spring or distilled water. As for distilled water, I learned you apply that to your iron when need steam. Springwater interacts with the supplements I take. Why? Good question. However, I would have your water tested because it could play a major role when you are taking medications or supplements.

How much I hate to say this. Do avoid caffeine. I love cappuccinos, caramel frappes, and citric fruits. You can get your iron from food sources. Make sure you get plenty of rest, massages twice a month, and modified exercise that support the muscles.

When I found out that I have lupus, I started searching on the internet, trying to figure out what was going on, what I had, and why. All I saw was you can die in your sleep, you could die, and there was no cure. That scared me, but I didn't hear much about what was being done about the disease. A lot of people didn't know much about lupus, and you don't hear anything about it on TV or radio stations. People hear more about saving animals, cancer, and children in other countries but nothing about lupus. Please understand, I have a dog, family members that has or had cancer and if I could, I would save the world. I also used to work with less fortunate children, and I placed my heart and soul into that job. So please do not take my statement the wrong way.

It was a terrifying feeling. I had sleepless nights and was very confused. Still, I began to dig more to figure out what lupus is and listen to other stories on blogs and other foundations websites. I also joined the Lupus Foundation of America to see how they were helping people. I found that my living conditions in my past could have exposed me to anything. But one thing you should know is that lupus is very hard to diagnose because it can appear to be just a chronic migraine, irritable bowel syndrome, chronic fatigue, Graves' disease, or rheumatoid arthritis, just to name a few. All the different diseases can overlap with each other leaving you to be misdiagnosed.

Living with lupus matters, just like cancer matters. Lupus lives matter. You'll feel like you're in denial. Then you become stressed because you can't understand why you are fatigued and restless all the time. I do have to say that I went to every rheumatologist in my network in the cities of Denton, Frisco, and Plano, Texas, and did not find not one rheumatologist who helped me. They did just enough for me to get by, and each one of the rheumatologists told me that they knew what they were doing because this was their profession and to trust them. I always ended up with the same information over again, mistakes, and less money in my pocket. One thing I would like for you to do so that you don't get the run-around is to get a full blood panel once a year because lupus does go dormant. Get tested for a C reactive protein, the sedimentation rate, a serum protein electro with a wrist sick, a standard CBC kick panel, and a complete blood count (CBC) with components such as a complete minute of C-3 and C-4 auto-antibodies, such as your anti-DNA, liver, and kidney functions just to name a few others.

Now that you know what lupus is and you understand the symptoms, you can bring awareness by telling someone what you read. Gift the book if you do not know how to explain the impact lupus plays in people lives. You can also help someone deal with what they may be going through or you are someone with lupus and can allow yourself to be the support system you need. People who you know and understand how this is affecting your life will be able to support you in your decisions regarding your healthcare and your lifestyle. There are going to be lots of times when you run across people who don't understand the reason why you choose not to eat meat or don't want to shake their hand or may be wearing a mask on your face. But they'll get over it. As far as pain management is concerned, do a generous workout if you feel like your pain is in control. Never work out if you cannot handle the pain, when you are light-headed, or when it's too hot or cold. If you are okay but not your legs, then just pick up a gallon of water and moving it up and down a few times while sitting in a chair. Do floor exercises. If your legs are okay and not your arms, then walk up and down some stairs a few times. A little motion is better than no motion at all. Make sure that you get your exercise in daily. It is very important to control pain. I know it sounds contrary because you're consistently in pain, but you've got to fight through it. You must get your exercise every day, making sure your diet and nutrition is on point.

THE IMMUNE SYSTEM

YOU CAN EXPLAIN this section to your family and friends so they can better understand what you are going through daily. Let's talk about the immune system. You've heard the phrase, *"You are what you eat."* Well, I have a new one: *"You are what you put on."* With my body, that is right. Have you ever looked at what is in your nail polish, soap, toothpaste, deodorant, perfumes, lotions, shampoo, and even chemicals, like perms and relaxers, you are putting in your hair? Well, all these things affect your immune system in some way. Yes, that's right, I said it! I am very guilty of a few things just mentioned. I want you to think about what I just said, and I will also explain to you some more research that I have done about our immune systems.

Now, remember, you are reading this book to learn about the autoimmune system, so I hope you are using posted notes or bookmarking your pages.

Let me define what the immune system is, according to a very prestigious hospital, John Hopkins (John Hopkins Lupus Center of America.com). John Hopkins lupus center clarifies that the immune system is *"an intricate network of cells, tissues, and organs that aids to guard your body against invaders like bacteria, viruses, fungal infections, and parasites."* Usually, the immune system grows only to act upon foreign elements, and immune system cells that try to battle with your body and are cleared out during the growth process. However, in lupus and other autoimmune diseases, the immune system begins to identify and attack itself. Yes, you read that correctly. Each cell is battling it out with each other. In other words, the cells of the immune system start to hurt the body's own tissue.

This experience can cause everlasting scarring that ultimately endangers the function of certain organs and systems in your body.

I want people from all walks of life to understand this book. Let me explain what an antibody is. What do they do for your body?

Antibodies are proteins that the body produces to protect itself from alien invaders, such as bacteria or viruses (WebMD.com)

Just as I broke down the T cells, let me tell you about another cell called lymphocytes. Lymphocytes include cells called B-cells and their job is to flag and fight infections in healthy individuals. Antigens are substances that provoke the response of T-cells and B-cells in the body. Just like a brawl, here come cytokines that then cause B-cells to multiply, and some of these B-cells turn into plasma cells that secrete antibodies (immunoglobulins). To provide an example, the response of B cells is signified as the humoral response. T-cell stimulation is called the cell-mediated immune response. Both antibodies then travel in the bloodstream so that when they meet the antigen again. T-Cell connects and forms a complex that is then replaced by other cells of your immune system to abolish the invader. Next, the remains of these complexes are detached from the body by a garbage disposal system that involves your spleen. Well, should I get a new spleen? Will that be a cure? Doctors, can you check into making new spleens? Lol, I would not be surprised if they don't have fake spleens. Soon we will have flying cars.

T-cells are classified as killer T-cells. I know that sounds bad, but killer T-cells can identify and destroy infected cells in the body. Bring it on, killer Ts, Yes, now if I could have "a cup a day, that would keep the infection away". I like that. I think I am going to patent this phrase.

Killer T-cells, however, can only recognize viruses flooded by extraordinary cells called macrophages. The macrophage presents the antigen to the killer -T cell, which responds by producing the cytokines that stimulate B-cells to increase and discharge antibodies.

In healthy individuals, the multitudes of cells that gather at an infected or injured site in the body produce factors that help fight off the infection. This process causes some inflammation and injury of healthy tissue, but usually, the immune system recollects other factors that help to control this inflammatory development. As for me or in individuals with lupus, both B-cells and T-cells become overactive. The two main concerns increased activity are the makings of autoantibodies (antibodies that recognize and destroy the body's own cells) and inflammation that can lead to long-term, irreversible destruction.

The making of autoantibodies in me or folks with lupus and other autoimmune diseases causes the immune system to aim toward the body's own cells for damage. For example, about 98 percent of people with lupus have antinuclear antibodies (ANA), which can attack the nucleic sector of your cells. In addition, some individuals may have antiphospholipid antibodies, which harm proteins bound to phospholipids in the membranes of your cells. These autoantibodies are linked to strokes, heart attacks, and blood clots. In addition, regulatory T-cells, which are supposed to control the structure, are lacking in SLE.

Am I taking too long to explain things? Good! Because this way, the more you know, the more you can explain and bring awareness. Next, you have neutrophils. Neutrophils are said to be the most common type of white blood cell in your body. Whereas lymphocytes are involved in the ongoing immune response, neutrophils are the first line of attack against invaders. Now! I need a tall on the invaders and venti on the whipped cream of neutrophils. Get it Starbucks Lol so much on my jokes.

Inflammation in a healthy individual usually signals that the body's immune system is reacting appropriately to pathogens, damaged cells, pain, or injury. However, with me, neutrophils caused increased inflammation due to certain connections between my blood plasma and other immune system cells (specifically, cytokines, and cell adhesion molecules). Even though increased inflammation may cause pain and discomfort, my major problem with inflammation is possible long-term irreversible damage. It is important that you and your doctor(s) or as for me naturopathic doctor discuss medications or supplements to control the inflammatory progressions involved in lupus to reduce long-term damage to vital organs. Some people with lupus and similar autoimmune diseases have a greater ratio of pro-inflammatory to anti-inflammatory cytokines than normal individuals, which produces an unbalanced controlling system.

While a general cause-and-effect connection between cytokines and lupus is not yet understood, certain cytokines called interferons and interleukins are related to the disease. In general, too many such molecules cause the immune system to become overexcited, leading to increased inflammation and tissue injury.

Supplement proteins interact in a progressive way to clear immune complexes from your body. In addition, since balance proteins are expended during inflammatory processes, low balance levels may imply lupus activity. This means you are now having a flare-up. Read more about flare-ups in part 2 of my book *Does CBD & MARIJUANA Help Lupus*.

GOD PLEASE HELP ME

NOW THAT YOU have a better understanding of what lupus is, what causes lupus, and why genetics can be important to lupus, allow me to touch "on a few" things people go though as for what I call "a journey". Millions of Americans have experienced an autoimmune disease. If this is you or someone you know, keep reading. You will be surprised by what you learn.

The reason I am writing this book because there are very few people in this world who share their journey about lupus. The word *lupus* is loosely used because, as I explained in the beginning, there are two types. When I found out I had lupus, the first thing I did was to search the internet to see how long I was going to live. I could not wait to go to the bookstore, thinking I could find books on an autoimmune disease that talked about the steps you would go through in your daily life. I found that most information found was not true because everyone's autoimmune disease reacts differently, and there are different symptoms for each person. So, I decided to get closer to God for understanding.

As I attach God to my journey, I went through a grieving period. One in every thousand people may go through the grieving process. There are five stages, some people will not go through them all in the order I have placed them but as for me, I went through each one noted below.

> I can do all things through him who strengthens me.
> (Philippians 4:13)

*My first stage was **Denial***: It started with not believing that I was sick. I did not tell anyone until I knew what to tell them. When learning about the stages of grief, I found that most people will experience this stage when first diagnosed. I can remember my aunt would come over to my apartment, open the curtains, and tell me to get up. My room would be the coldest place in the apartment. I would refuse her every time, and she would have to force me out of bed or trick me by offering something. She would tell me all the time that I was a vampire. My house stayed clean all but my bedroom. I would have things everywhere. The most important thing you need to understand that this is important to know this is a natural reaction. I was likely overwhelmed with what I had learned and block out the many facts I read like I was going to die. Some people may be better equipped to deal with the initial shock. However, I spent the first three years of my illness at this stage. Knowing about this chronic illness, finally came to the realization that I needed help, like counseling. I was advised that this stage can be detrimental, as I could pretend the illness does not exist and therefore would not finally seek the medical treatment I needed. I was noncompliant with medication, skipped doctor appointments to save money, and would talk about death all the time telling my family to "just put me in a wood box or cremate me" I did not care. I was done.

Have you ever found yourself simply closing your eyes and wishing the pain would go away? I certainly know I have. Denial can be a devastating position. I know this from personal experience. I remember going to Chicago with my sister, and I went to a picnic in the park. When I made it to the park, the smell of food, smoke, and old water (Lake Michigan) was making me feel abnormal. I was having symptoms as if I were pregnant. I ignored the symptoms for as long as I could. I told my sister that I needed to leave. She was not happy about that because she drove and had to take me back to where we were staying. I messed her day up. After resting a few hours, I was fine, but I did not know why I was feeling so strange. Now she doesn't ask me out anymore unless I am driving by myself. I did not want to talk to anyone. My smile was not real. All I could think about was laying down.

Another time, I remember driving to San Antonio with my husband for one of my anniversaries, and we stayed at a hotel on the Riverwalk. When we left the hotel and walked on the path of the river, I began to feel sick. I then asked my husband to take me back to the hotel because I did not feel good. After sleeping for a few hours, I felt better. However, everything was closed, so we ended up going home and I ruined the trip. When I made it back home, I ended up at the hospital. My lab numbers were very high. Something was wrong. My doctor didn't seem to take my condition too seriously, so I certainly did not think I needed too. He advised it was just a form of arthritis and we would follow up in six weeks. Well, not quite. In my mind, I didn't really have much to worry about. I didn't think it was a big deal. When I think back now, I realize that it may have been a necessary process for coming to terms with my illness. After I spoke with my doctors, no one could explain why I get sick when traveling. At this point in my life, I don't want to leave the state because it does not matter where I go. I get sick.

At any rate, I continued down the same path of denial. My life was right where I wanted it. I have an advanced degree and planned to excel by opening my own business until I retire. I am a mother and had a lot on my plate. Like many others, I was not accustomed to putting my needs anywhere near the top of the list. Other things were far more important, or at least that is what I thought, and it worked for me for a while.

Yet he was merciful, he forgave their iniquities and did not destroy them, Time after time he restrained his anger and did not stir up his full wrath. (Psalm 78:38)

*My second stage was **Anger***: Everyone has experienced anger at one time or another, and those with chronic illnesses are no exception. Some people will argue that anger is one of the most common emotions that humans are most familiar with when dealing with lupus. As for me, it seems to almost be a needed stage in my healing process because it allows me to discover the depths of my feelings and get them out in the open.

The anger I felt was primarily towards myself; however, it eventually extended to family, friends, and even the medical community that delivered the overwhelming news or who wanted to provide treatment. I found myself saying, "This isn't fair!" I was questioning God, I hated. my mother, and my father for making me, "What did I do to deserve this?" playing sad songs was my favorite, talking about people that looked happy all the time was my forte.

The anger I felt was irrational at times, but I allowed my attitude to take over. Cry and scream every day to do what is necessary to cope, but I was never willing to be open to my counselors or family who were there to help me through this stage.

> Come to me, all who labor and are heavy laden, and I will give you rest. (Matthew 11:28)

I followed with **Bargaining**: Just as the name implies, this is when I found myself attempting to strike a deal with God, a higher power, or even the doctors who were committed to my care. This is also a stage of "if only" or "what if" statements, and I found myself dealing with feelings, I took my life and health seriously like I was told to do by my family. What if, we were rich? Would that have made a difference in my life? It goes on!

After dealing with anger and foolish thoughts, bargaining was my attempt at rationalizing the situation and regaining control. Certainly, I wanted to protect myself from the pain of my new reality and the unchartered territory of my condition, but ultimately my purpose here seems to be asking lupus please go away don't ruin my life. "Don't take me now, Lord, I will do what you ask of me". I had so many plans, but as the days went by, it became more real that I had to deal with this situation of pain every day. I still would cry out in the shower, get on my knees before I go to bed "begging" "Let me live, Lord, I will act right. I will not be mad at the world. I want to live to see my children have children. Please, Lord, give me a chance".

Of course, I was willing to do anything to have the situation change, or at least that was one of the things I wished to proclaim. This readiness' to do anything was not completely realistic, but it motivated me to continue counseling.

> Casting all your anxieties on him, because he cares for you. (1 Peter 5:7)

During counseling, she advised me I was in the **Depression** *stage*: Although the stage of bargaining was my motivation to continue counseling, the depressive stage paused that motivation in its tracks. As the reality of my condition set in, I was becoming overwhelmed with feelings of helplessness, a sense of void and sadness. I was feeling all alone. However, the counselor advised me that this is a natural response to feeling like you have no soul, and or life and chronic illness is certainly a thrashing. It was the absence of what my life once was before I found out I had lupus.

You might find yourself withdrawn during this *stage*, as I did. There were times when I wondered, "What's the point? I'm going to be sick forever, so why bother fighting?" It is important to know that these were normal feelings, and I could not let them control my viewpoint on life. However, for years I was not able to complete goals, I was from job to job or on a form of assistant to make sure I had medical insurance. However, depression never left, and I could not see life the same again. My family now sees something is wrong and have questions. I had to tell but at that stage I was in, I did not believe they were much help.

Often with depression comes anxiety. I found myself worrying about insurance, medical bills, social situations, making sure I had makeup for my face when going out into the public, my inability to live up to expectations for work, not wanting a boyfriend anymore and of course nothing to do with God's plan. I went to church but would do the opposite of what was being taught. Do not have sex outside of marriage. Well, here comes the babies. I had so much anxiety that nothing in life was going right. I gained weight, every business I tried to open failed, going to school took forever and my relationships all the way up to marriage was hard, because I could not be open to what was going on with my body.

I found that being open and honest about these feelings helped me battle the journey of depression and anxiety. Being depressed or feeling anxious does not mean you are unstable or mentally ill. When I was experiencing these feelings, it was to express the necessary steps to healing. To work on me and find my way back to God. We are human, and those around you may understand your feelings better than you realized. I found that out as I accepted my invader.

> For if their rejection brought reconciliation to the world,
> what will their acceptance be but life from the dead?
> (Romans 11:15)

As I completed my time with the counselor, I was at the *Acceptance stage*: This stage was the crucial goal, yet I believe it is greatly misinterpreted. Accepting lupus does not mean that I was suddenly okay with being sick. I was not convinced that it is even possible! I do not think I will ever get to the point of thinking it is all right to carry this disease with no cure; however, I can acknowledge the reality of my illness and come to terms with myself to set goals on bringing awareness before I die.

For some, this is a peaceful state and an opportunity to find new enjoyment in life. The reality of the situation is, I am sick, and my life looks different than it did before or what my plan is no more but that does not mean my life no longer has a purpose. Thoughts of having acceptances, I was able to find a new outlook on life. However, I made modifications and gained a better understanding of what I will be faced with moving forward.

Going through the stages provided me a renewed spirit and a willingness to battle to the end. I have become knowledgeable about my illness, I work out regularly, and I take supplements appropriately. I eat very little meat if any at all, and I make sure that I am stress-free. I have a lot to live for, and I appreciate every day as a small victory.

Lupus is a condition I have, but it does not define who I am. By ultimately accepting my new life, I have a greater appreciation for all it has to offer. As a result, an abundance of learning and growing opportunities has risen that I would never have experienced otherwise, and I am grateful each day. One good thing is I have embraced who I am, and all I have to offer to others in life is love and knowledge. Recognize that you are an amazing person, and take the opportunity to spread lupus awareness by given to lovelifelupusfoundation.org to help others. By doing this, you can effectively bring meaning to the lives of people with this disease and potentially find that acceptance is a far more desirable stage to bear.

In the end, the process of grief is not limited to death. It also affects those with chronic illnesses or those going through a similar process.

All five stages may not be practiced in the same order of the stages that I went through. However, the goal and the final stage is acknowledgment. It can be challenging to adequately deal with your illness until this final stage is completed.

(SOME) OF THE SYMPTOMS YOU GO THROUGH

AFTER GOING THROUGH what I thought where the devil lies, I found that I will not bash any physicians. I think about all the money that was spent visiting different doctors and taken over 15 different medications and receiving no results. Having lupus is very tiring. You feel fatigued or like you have the flu 90 percent of the time. I want to nap all day, which then leads to insomnia and or anemia. My energy level is always low unless you add sugar in your life which feeds, the invaders. My bed becomes my best friend.

Anemia, yes! having a nosebleed, heavy cycles put my sex life now downhill. After acquiring from Mayo Clinic, the clinic defines been anemia as a condition in which you don't have enough healthy red blood cells to carry enough oxygen to the body's tissues. What is next? If I don't have enough oxygen to the body's tissues, will I stop breathing? No! but was advised to take medication that is either provided by a doctor or over the counter. Do you know what happens next? Well, I then became constipated because I had too much iron. Iron is a mineral that's necessary for life. Iron plays a key role in the making of red blood cells, which carry oxygen. I was told that I have an iron deficiency but never was told what the side effects are.

Make sure you ask. As for me, it was causing an upset stomach, and the worst of it all chronic constipation. When I talked to the doctors about constipation, all they could do was take me off the iron pills or provide something for constipation. Wow!

As for me, I headed to the gastroenterologist, which led to surgery. No laxative could help. After a few months after surgery, it started all over again. When I went back to my primary physician, he did lots of blood work and tests, but nothing could explain the pain, migraines, fatigue, and skin spots on my face, arms, chest, and back. All he could say was it could have stemmed from my upbringing or could be hereditary.

Let me mention again about my upbringing. For the first time, I thought a doctor was right. This could be the only way I can validate how in some form lupus is related. I did a lot of moving, but a change in my life took place when I moved back to Texas. Things were going well until I was introduced to a big blow called a stroke. Now I have a hearing problem and I am partially blind. What's next?

STROKE, STROKE, GO AWAY, DON'T COME BACK ANOTHER DAY

A song called "A Night to Remember" by Shalamar is my jam. This is a day to remember. I was living on my own and had my first beautiful baby girl (Ki-Ki). She is the joy of my life. I realized that I did not know what real love was until she was born. I was working two jobs. My sister was living with me and had a beautiful baby girl also (Kelli-Wellie). I came home with the girls from picking them up from daycare, and my sister was cooking dinner as she still loves to do today so I decided to give the girls a bath. The bathwater was made, and I put them in the tub. We were singing nursery songs, and I was dancing. Next thing I knew, I was in the hospital in ICU and could not move the left side of my body.

I had a stroke and was paralyzed on the left side of my body. The doctors said that it was stress. I could not walk for months. All my friends were gone. I had no job and was very sad. My family was very supportive. My uncle came from Chicago on his birthday to stay and help. However, I was blessed to recover after a year. The thing about this stroke was that the doctors could not understand the recovery and the fact that I was so young. I never did ask how that affected my sister, and the girls were too young to remember. However, this changed my outlook on life forever.

The doctors could not find a reason for me to have such a major health problem at a young age. However, the doctors felt that the diagnosis of the stroke came from stress. I was paralyzed on the left side of my body for twelve months and ten days and recovered very well. God is good. Over the years, after having the stroke I would get the flu or a cold every other month. I started to get E. coli twice a month. Doctors could not explain why, but my family advised that I would need to keep things a lot cleaner in my home and my car and change my eating habits. My health was not getting better, and doctors still could not explain it. All they would say was, "You are a young lady your body will heal in time." All your tests are negative, and this issue will pass. Take this can call me in two weeks for a follow-up. So, what I would gather out of that, it's all in my head.

Well, time moved on, and I started to have more children. With all three of my children, I could not work during my pregnancy because I was considered a high-risk patient. My blood cell numbers would be normal, and they would run test after test. Still, nothing could be explained. At this point, I would just deal with it. This would cause issues with my job because it would seem as if I did not want to work. I would get the flu and would go to work and was not able to perform at 100 percent.

This went on for years and as time went by, I began to have more pain. The doctor had me on conventional medicine that was not working. That led to me seeing other doctors, and no one could provide an answer. Again, a doctor stated after taking my blood, "I am sorry to tell you, you have Graves' disease." Graves' disease, what next, also known as toxic diffuse goiter, which is an autoimmune disease that affects the thyroid. It also causes swelling of the neck and protrusion of the eyes, resulting from an overactive thyroid gland. Another word for it is an exophthalmic goiter.

In the mid-nineteenth century, a man named Robert J. Graves (1796–1853) was an Irish physician who first identified Graves' disease. This immune system disorder of the butterfly-shaped gland in the throat (thyroid) can be treated by an anti-thyroid medication, radioactive iodine, to help restore the thyroid function to normal. However, the thyroid-encouraging antibodies cause the Graves' disease to revert. With all the side effects, I decided to leave the thyroid untreated, which caused serious problems with my heart, bones, muscles, and at the time, my menstrual cycle. I decided to seek another opinion. I was always referred to the best doctor in town to the point where I would drive for hours to get help.

The first thing I said God has sent me another sign, "Oh, it's time to die. Let me get myself together and fix all the wrong that has been done." Let me find all the people I know and say I am sorry for what I have said or done to you. I felt I needed to do that so that I can heal on the inside before it was my time to die. My symptoms got worse, with irritability, muscle weakness, and sleeping problems. I could not go out into the sun, missing my children's outdoor sports events, and I had a fast heartbeat that keeps me from talking for a long period of time, no tolerance of heat, and wow not to mention the up-and-down weight loss. I said to myself, "Lord, just take me now." Well, God did not take me, and I was taken medication for years, and the only thing that was changing was my skin tone. It was time to see a dermatologist.

I went to doctor after doctor, had skin grafts done, and got lots of topical treatments and soaps, and nothing. My face started to get more white spots, and no doctor could explain why but "call me in two weeks for a follow up appointment". The top dermatologist in Texas, who was famous for working with stars like Michael Jackson, treated me for two years, and now my bills were starting to grow. The only thing that was changing was the money in my pocketbook.

I would smell like burnt fried chicken every time I got out of the spaceship (when having my treatments done). After an evaluation, I was advised to take more medication and have six more months of chemotherapy. I did not have good insurance, so I had to pay out of pocket each time I went to see the doctor, along with paying for the tolls, gas, and parking. Next, the doctor I was seeing at the time advised me after an additional six months of treatment to do another year of chemotherapy. At that point, I felt that I was been tested on like they do rats, and I declined the services. Suddenly, the nurse said, "Have a great day, Mrs. Bias. See you same time tomorrow."

As I was running out of the hospital on the way to the parking lot, I got into my car and went to pay the parking guard. My heart was racing faster than normal. Before I knew it, I screamed "No, no, no! Why me?"

I became fed up. Enough was enough. As I was crying, I felt I needed to call my grandmother, whom I love so much, and told her, "Grandma, I cannot do this. I can't continue to go to the doctors and leave feeling like a test dummy and smell like burnt chicken. The doctors really don't know what's wrong with me. They can't give me a diagnosis. The doctors never come and see me after I come out of the roasted chicken bend. I see them twelve times a month, and there is no change. They can't tell me what's going on, and I want to know why."

My grandmother took a deep, deep breath. Then she said, "It's okay, baby. In time they will find out." I was screaming my lungs out, I didn't have time.

At that point, I wanted to take my car and drive it off the road. However, the sound of my grandmother's voice as she spoke to me was so different after she heard my statement. For the first time in my life, I found that my grandmother was scared and all she could do is tell me that she did not want any of her children dying before her. She proceeded to calm me down by telling me that she loved me and that I was no different than any other person because I was loved. I know she was praying for me in her head because she was not with me in the car as I yelled out for help. Help Me Please, Help me, Please, grandma please. She just told me things were going to be okay as her voice crackled very softly. My grandmother, who is a senior citizen, would always say that she knew I would live longer than her. All she could do was cry with me and say she was sorry. At that moment, I think she was hurt because there was nothing that she could do for me.

She asked me not to give up but to just go see another doctor. Still, I was not convinced. I told my grandmother that I loved her, and I would talk with her soon. She asked me not to do anything that would not get me into heaven. I explained that I was done. No more being tested like a rat. No more being their test dummy. I am so DONE!

My grandmother said, "Well, before you do anything, please call your aunt (she is like a mother to me) and tell her how you feel." I told her no because she was going to say the same thing. My grandmother got mad and said, *"Now, Tonya. Call her now!"*

When she said that, something just came over me, and I said, *"Yes, Mama."* I called my aunt and said, "Help me," as I was crying. She said, "Pull the car over first, and I will talk to you." I said NO she stated then call me back when you do. I said ok, I am pulling over. I did as she said, and she started praying. She must have heard the sadness in my voice that I could not deal with this disease anymore. This prayer was so deep that no words can describe how I felt afterward. All I know is my life was changing at that moment and I could not give up because I was reminded I am here for a purpose.

OB-GYN WHY?

AS THE YEARS go by, time for an annual checkup with my Ob-gyn. During the checkup, I explained that I stop seeing doctors because no one could find out why I am in so much pain all the time and why my skin produces white spots. Along, with being in and out of the hospitals for fatigue. The recommendation, which never failed when it comes to traditional doctors was lots of blood taken. This time the reason was due to being in and out of the hospitals for pain and fatigue, and no one could find out what was wrong. The results are in; Well, Latonya, I must tell you the news. We cannot find anything all the tests came back negative. Work to change your diet because you are overweight. However, for them to be safe it was once again "Referral time". The ob-gyn referred me to another rheumatologist. This was not something I wanted to do and at this point, I was $200,000 in debt of medical bills, plus my joints, muscles, and ligaments in my body had me in so much pain I must get people to drive me around. I could not take pain medication because it would put me to sleep and I would not be able to work.

The ob-gyn stated, "I am not a specialist in pain, and I hear that is what you complain a lot about. Your numbers are low, you keep getting E. coli, and we cannot find a cause." I was always tired and fatigued when I went anywhere, so I gave it a try. I was overweight but I kept saying I was done with doctors. Friends and family would say "you cannot be done with doctors until you find out what was going on with you." I called my rock. She explained that it would not hurt to go, so I went.

These three doctors advised the same thing: "You have lupus."

I was screaming at the top of my lungs. When I asked doctors what to do, I was advised that I would have to take medication for the rest of my life since there was no cure. Now the real journey would begin. Before my eyes could blink, I was in the world of medication I called it "pill city". I was taking medication for an inflammatory condition, arthritis, headaches, my heart, my joints and muscles, fatigue, my bladder, runny eyes, bowel problems, infection after infection, and then some. It seems like the side effects made things worse, and doctors would add more prescriptions.

I felt like I was suppressing symptoms. I am not trying to discredit the work of doctors, but I can say from experience that I have been through a lot of doctors, and none have worked out for me. I was anxious and stressed to the point where I had to file for FLMA because I needed to take off work when it was to cold, hot or raining. I told my husband I could not live in a cold or hot environment due to my health. I could not travel for longer than three hours in a car or to other states. I could not go on boats so I need to find another state to live in because I would not make it here in Texas. Hello, world. Then come the sunshine and heat. Wow, again, I just needed to live in a bubble.

My main doctor was not sure if I had lupus because what I did find out is that when your numbers are good then you are in remission, so lupus will not show up, but if a flare-up takes place and you go get blood work done, the test will come back with lupus or an autoimmune disease.

I went to an immune specialist (a hematologist, another name is a blood doctor). They deal with problems with the red blood cells, white blood cells, platelets, blood vessels, bone marrow, lymph nodes, spleen, and the proteins involved in bleeding and clotting (hemostasis and thrombosis). A hematologist applies his specialized knowledge to treat me. When I spoke with the hematologist, my reason for going was to find out why I kept getting bacterial infections. All that doctor told me was, "Everything looks good. I need you to take iron pills." Well, guess what? If I took iron pills, it would cause constipation. If I had constipation, then I would not be able to pass stool, which will lead me back to the gastroenterologist. What a cycle. I went back to the gastroenterologist to check for celiac disease and ended up leaving the doctor's office with a set appointment for minor surgery. This experience did not go too well again.

The doctor did the surgery. I woke up from the surgery to hear my doctor tell me, "You are just fine. Check back in a year for a follow-up."

Not, "Just want to let you know the reason that we are doing this surgery is to…" or "What I did will help in this way because…" I received no results, and I did not go back. I fault myself on this one because I did not ask any questions before I had surgery. The doctor made it out to be a part of the checkup. It was the end of the year and he wanted money which was out-of-pocket for the surgery before my insurance would start over with co-pay.

The whole approach is based on getting to the root of the problem, but as I continued to cry to family, it was explained that I need to change my eating habits and go see a naturopathic doctor. I think it's time! I stopped eating meat except for chicken but found that it was not enough. I was having a lot of side effects, and I was not getting better. I was getting worried.

Naturopathic doctors are educated and trained in accredited naturopathic medical colleges. They diagnose, prevent, and treat acute and chronic illnesses to restore and establish optimal health by supporting the person's inherent self-healing process. Rather than just suppressing symptoms, naturopathic doctors work to identify underlying causes of illnesses and develop personalized treatment plans to address them. The way they work identifies the natural order in which all therapies should be applied to provide the greatest benefit with the least potential for damage.

One day I had a bad experience with a naturopathic doctor. I am not saying to give one a try because in the end, I found a good one. However, I need to tell you this crazy story. I had been asking around at work if anyone knew a good naturopathic doctor who was reasonable. One of my coworkers who looked like a crackhead told me that she had cataracts. She went to see a naturopathic doctor, and after six months, she was healed of cataracts. My coworker provided me the number, and I called and set up an appointment. I spoke with a lady on the phone who sounded very young and was very upbeat. She only asked for my phone number and provided me a date and time to come in.

She said, "I will see you soon, sweetie."

I found her to be very nice and outgoing. Then I realized that I did not give her my name. I attempted to call back a few times, and the voicemail stated, "You have reached a number that has been disconnected."

As time went by, I did not think anything of it and just planned on going to see the highly recommend a naturopathic doctor. Naturopathic doctors are not covered under insurance. I found out later why they don't take insurance. Hopefully, I will have an answer in my next book part 2 *Does CBD & MARIJUANA Help Lupus.* As I was on my way to my appointment, my navigation system took me to an old, abandoned building. Next door was the doctor's office. As I started walking to the door, I could smell an unwanted aroma. I have a big nose, and to me, it smelled like old, smelly feet. As I rang the doorbell, I was let in and had to walk down a long hall. Walking down this hall felt like it took forever. I made it to the door and was greeted by a very fragile woman with long gray hair down her back. Her face had holes all in her cheeks. My first thought was *Run. Get out as fast as you can. I am in a scary movie.* But I could not move.

She spoke very slow and said, "Welcome. Are you Tonya? Have a seat, my dear."

Oh no, I think I have a situation. I slowly moved to sit down in a chair that looks like if I sat my big but on it, I was going to hit the floor. As I slowly looked for the door, it seemed so far away. Now I was scared first because I did not tell the lady on the phone my name, and second, the place had old jars with brown stuff and water in them on the counter. I asked the lady her name, and she acted like she did not hear me. I asked the name of the place to see if I was in the right location, and she stated, "Yes, dear, you are."

I did not feel well. My stomach started to hurt, my left eye was watering, and the smell of the place had me putting my lips up over my nose. Before I knew it, I quickly pulled out my phone and pretended to look at it as if I had a text and told the lady that I had to go. I could not move fast enough as I get to the door, and when I pulled on it, it would not open. I pulled a second time, and again it would not open. Well, the old lady had to buzz me out. How did I miss that coming in?

I said to the lady, "Is something wrong with the door?"

I was trying not to show fear as she said, "Wait a minute, dear."

After that, all I know is I was running down the hall and was in my car within seconds. I returned to work the next day and told my coworkers what happened. I asked my coworker about the location and the lady. My coworker said she did not know what I was talking about, as if I had gone to the wrong address. I felt like my coworker was playing a trick on me. I confirmed the address and phone number with her because now I feel like this is a game my co-worker was doing. Later that day, I decided to drive back to the address since it was not wrong per my co-worker. There were bars on the door as if no one had rented the space. The first thing I said was, "How could this be? I know I was in the right place." Later that month I found out that the building was where homeless people lived. All I can say is I am so happy I have two feet.

One of my family members has been going to a naturopathic doctor for years, and she has not been sick like most people. Health, the natural state of one's body, is disturbed by obstacles that lead to disease. I would hear, "Girl, the first step in returning to a good bill of health is to remove the entities that cause poor health, such as poor diet, digestive disorders, unsuitable and chronic stress levels, and individual conflict." So, I gave another naturopathic doctor a try.

NATUROPATHIC DOCTORS

NATUROPATHIC DOCTORS' IDEA of a healthy treatment is based on an individual's problems to health to modify and improve the grounds in which diseases are established. Well, what did that tell me? I needed to try it again. If I can take natural treatments without side effects, I am in. I found a real naturopathic doctor to interview and answer a few questions. The naturopathic doctor in Texas explained that she uses therapies to stimulate and strengthen the body's innate self-healing and healing skills. These therapies are comprised of modalities such as clinical nutrition, plant-based supplements, hydrotherapy, homeopathy, and acupuncture. Also, it enhances precise tissues, organs, or systems, including lifestyle involvements, dietary changes, and orthomolecular therapy used for materials that happen naturally in the body, such as vitamins, amino acids, and minerals.

This time, I asked lots of questions, but needed to know "Do they use the same therapy or treatments for the same healing issues?" The answer to this question was, "No." People who have the same issues are addressed with a different level of a healing process. This was because each person's body build is different from weight, age, and symptoms.

While many naturopathic doctors are trained in primary care, like conventional medical doctors (MDs), some choose to specialize or focus on their own practices. I was advised that naturopathic medical education programs include certain areas of study not covered in conventional medical school. At the same time, aspiring naturopathic doctors receive training in the same biomedical and diagnostic sciences as MDs and osteopathic doctors (DOs).

The result is a full, severe, and well-rounded scientific medical education that is both similar and balancing to that of MDs and DOs. You can see why I was asking a lot of questions, and even after finding a good naturopathic doctor, I was still skeptical. I started using both medication and plant base supplements because I was scared to let the medication go. However, over time, I slowly took myself off the doctor's recommendation medication and started the process with a great naturopathic doctor. You should talk with all your doctors first because what happened to me next can happen to you.

One Sunday morning, I was not feeling well enough to go to church, so my family went without me. What I am about to explain happen before I started to see a naturopathic doctor. After services, they came home to pick me up so we could go out for breakfast. They came home to find me lying face-down and unconscious between the hall and the bedroom floor. I was not feeling good the night before and was restless. I was not sure what took place, yet, I woke up in the hospital. The doctors were not sure what was wrong and why I was unconscious, so they treated me with medication as if I was having a flare-up from my lupus.

I was provided pain medication, something for the swelling, blood thinner, lupus medication, and a few other things, which they called a "cocktail". I was sent home from the hospital and was advised to stay off my feet for a few days. Let me mention that they did find blood clots in my right leg, but nothing was done about it.

My husband felt that I was taking too much medication and wanted me to find another doctor to help me limit the number of meds I was taking. When I did that, I ended up receiving more because they ran tests and something else was wrong. At that point, he wanted me to stop looking for doctors and work out and eat healthier. He did not want me to take any of the medications if he had to worry about leaving me at home alone.

I received a letter in the mail from the hospital explaining that my blood work came back. It turned out that it was a flare-up. Every time I had a flare-up, which could be two or three times a month depending on the situation and what season it was, I ended up resting, depending on prayers, or going to the hospital to get a "cocktail".

Next, I had a panic attack, and insomnia kicked in. I felt as though I was living in a prison of dizziness and fatigue. I did not want to go anywhere or do anything, not even the hospital. The bills were piling up. I would go to work and come home and get into bed. My social life took a hit, and my sex life left me with cobwebs downtown. The spots on my face became bigger, and they were now spreading further down my back and legs. I had no energy. No, no, no, my health was now out of control.

I could not believe this was happening to me. I started thinking about all the things I needed to do and if I would have the time to do them. How was I going to tell my children, and would they understand? Because right now all they saw was their mother working and sleeping. I couldn't attend any football games, which I hated because that was a big part of my sons' lives. I couldn't attend any basketball games, and those were a big part of my daughter's life. I had to stay out of the sun because it would make me feel weak and dizzy, and my mood swings were shot. No family vacations. Now I was stressed. I could not help around the house, and my children felt like I did nothing. I began to feel like I was becoming a failure as a mom, wife, and friend.

Food started to become a part of my life and not in a good way. I was eating everything you can think of, from four to five pieces of chicken (dark meat) to drinking one or two-liters of pop/soda (Coke) and big bags of chips and cookies (peanut butter), not to mention two bags chocolate and caramel-covered clusters of peanuts by myself. Part of that was due to the medication I was taking. With all the medication, the diet went out the door. I had a leaky gut, toxins and infections became my new friend.

The routines did not go away, and when I would look at myself in the mirror, I was convinced I needed to do something. Let start with all the weight-loss programs. After thousands of dollars spent, I could have saved and had a brand-new car because that was a waste of money. Next, I tried no fried foods, which did not work. What about eating salads and vegetables? Well, that helped a little, but over the years I was still the same weight and still had a lot of medications to take.

I was now at the point, since I had developed an autoimmune condition, that the conventional medicines had failed me. I was at 210 pounds. Oh no, we have another situation. If you are one of the millions who struggle with an autoimmune disease, you may struggle with weight. It is always good to hear that someone else is on the same path as you. I am not saying like most books would say, "Read this book and it can change your life." I am going to be truthful about my life and how God has put me on a path of sharing my story called *Lupus: It Chose Me*.

I would always have heavy periods that would go for two to three weeks and lots of headaches. I never wanted to go anywhere because I was tired all the time. However, the family stepped in with lots of encouragement, and I was able to get back on my feet within a year.

You know what? There is something about God's love that just knocks you off your feet. I found that I was one of those people who would call on God when I needed him, and God would show up right on time. He never left me because I went through some tough times in my life. He has always let me know that I am his child of God.

One day I had a long day at work. I was very tired and weak and wanted to just lay down, but when I came home, there were other things to do around the house, with family, the dog, etc. It was late when I went to bed, but I was not that sleepy. As I was resting, my tongue started to itch. Then came a sharp pain. Now what? I got up, went into the bathroom, and looked at my tongue in the mirror. I thought, *Okay, I think we have another situation.* I could not close my mouth, or I would not be able to breathe. You know that the tongue is a muscular organ in the mouth and is used in the act of swallowing. I was not sure why, but I was having a hard time breathing. I was thinking about what I could have eaten that would cause my tongue to grow the size of a lemon. I waited and waited, thinking it was just me, and allowed hours to go by. However, it got to the point, I could feel my tongue getting bigger and bigger in my mouth. At the time my family only had one car, and my husband was gone to work. I did not know what to do. I could not talk, so I could not call 911. Thank God there was an emergency room down the street.

I walked to the emergency room and found out that I was having a mild stroke. I advised the doctors as I was slurring my words at three o'clock in the morning, I had lupus, and they looked as if they did not know what to do. I was left in the room for hours after taking the medication that they gave to take the swelling down. The doctors came back and asked what the hospital would give me if I was having a flare-up. I explained the cocktail, but they did not get it. The doctors came back and told me to follow up with my primary doctor. They told me the swelling should go down in a few hours, and if not, I should return to the emergency room. They told me, I was having a mini stroke and asked how I got to the hospital. I advised that I walked, the doctors looked at each other and one of them said "we are going to send you home, why did you walk, I explained.

I understood and called my rheumatologist the next day. She gave me a prescription for an EpiPen. The rheumatologist advised that I needed to keep the EpiPen on me always. After they ran blood work and lots of tests, it was found to be a stroke, but no one could tell me how it happened and what to do if it happens again. Enough is enough. I could not complete my goals in life or take the next steps to move forward because I kept having issues. Why? I don't know, and no doctor knows.

Now it's time to pay attention to the body. You only have one life to live and very few chances of doing it right. I know that life is about the choices you make, and I must look at my past to make sure I don't keep making the same mistakes. After many other episodes of swelling eyes, spitting up parasites, flare-ups, having blood clots the size of lemons, and waking up to my eyes closed shut, not because of a cold or flu, it was time to make a change.

That transformation put me in a path of a light workout and watching the types of foods I eat (no meat). Sometimes life can be very difficult if you don't pay attention to your body. If you don't listen, you find yourself in a very tough situation, wondering why you cannot put your wedding ring on, why one eye looks bigger than the other even with makeup on, or even why you aren't able to put shoes on.

To give you a little bit more of my history, we moved around a lot, living in low-income homes watching my mom go from job to job. My father was not around because he was serving his country. The grandmothers, aunts, and uncles stepped up to do what they could. However, I remember when I was nine years old, I was in pain and did not know why. I found myself struggling to go to sleep, so I had to count the cars out of the window and pray to become grown, thinking that all the pain would go away. I found myself moving too fast. I was hanging out late and finding things to get into. Life was showing me that life is like a box of chocolates, and you never know what you are going to get. I always found myself wondering what the next piece of my puzzle would be in life. I've been through so many changes in my life. I've seen and heard things. But I wonder what more can I see, what more can be lived.

I would go to church from time to time, thinking it would bring my grandmother back, but the words of the preacher and songs that were sung went right over my head. I felt like I had no purpose in life until I saw one of my family members leave Chicago to go to college. I was so mad because she was all I had. She was always full of life, smiling, and encouraging.

At that time, there were so many role models, but nothing stood out for me as she did. Music was in my ear, and the negativity of the streets was on my back. Now, where would I go for the love, attention, support, and guidance now that my grandmother was gone, and my family member was leaving? All of this was needed in my life. I was a sheep without a shepherd, and it was time for me to act on my life. What should I do? I could move out of my environment to another state. Maybe, a different part of the city. I don't know! This was very hard to grasp because I was not used to seeing diversity or change. Over time, moving was great because it helped me to defend myself and avoid judgment.

I found that my family line was not a healthy stock of people. They had cancer, multiple sclerosis, diabetes, heart failure, gout, and drug and alcohol addiction just to name a few. The ones I loved the most were passing away or coming up missing, placing me closer to God. Could this be the reason I am the way I am today? must think that God only knows.

> Jesus went throughout Galilee, teaching in the synagogues, announcing the good news of the kingdom, and healing every disease and sickness are among the individuals. Find a church home and the disciples can pray for you of any issues you may have, and the healing for every disease and sickness that comes upon you. (Matthew 4:23 NIV)

I found that to be my covenant. No matter how much pain you are in, you have prayed to stop the sadness and sickness of the heart. You will have to work twice as harder as healthy people to feel better, to be happy, along with being fulfilled with life. One important thing is the tree of life is special. Don't just talk about what you wish you could do. I know it is very hard to get up but try a little each day to get up and do something about what could be important to you in your life. Try not to make promises to yourself that you cannot keep. That is a set up for a bad comeback.

DOCTORS/ MEDICATION

SOME PEOPLE IN my family do not like doctors, so they will not go for help. When getting close to God the bible states "It is not the healthy people who need help but the sick" (Matthew 9:12). The best way to explain this quote is that there nothing wrong with doctors but do your research first and get second and third opinions until you feel you have the right doctor(s). As for me, I learned that going down the natural path works best. I am not at 100% but I am at 50% I am doing things that I have not been able to do in years. I am loving life and making sure that I am grateful every day I can see the sun, smell the roses, touch my children, and taste healthy food.

People want to know why I wrote this book. I want the world to know what happens when you get a disease that does not have any cure. I want the world to know that it has been an injustice from the doctors, the medication, testing, our environment, to the political situation in working on a cure. I want the world to know that autoimmune diseases are alive and working hard to take you down. I want the world to know that we must make a change about what to do when people do not understand that our lives are short and the only person you can lean on is our Father who is in heaven.

I created a lupus charity called Love Life Lupus Foundation Inc (lovelifelupusfoundation.org), which will help others understand how, who, what, when, where, why, when dealing with autoimmune diseases mainly lupus. The goal is to spread the word, allowing business and human resources to provide training, Doctors, other medical professionals, insurance companies, and the Social Security office to understand that people with autoimmune diseases need to become accommodated versus discriminated against. I also want people to understand that this book is not a prescription.

This book allows people to get and understand of what one person can go through with an autoimmune disease. I am not a medical professional. I am not a doctor. I am only a person who has gone through the tribulations of what is talked about in this book. I will be an advocate until the day I leave this earth.

The medications are going to be described in the following chapter. Please consult with your doctor before attempting to use any medication that is being discussed because all medications that are listed in this book are not good for everyone or what has been said is for everyone.

There's a prescription made out for each individual, so consult your doctors. I want this to be a guide to the understanding of one person's experience and to understand how much an autoimmune disease can affect a person's life. One would recommend seeing a naturopathic doctor. For this was the best way to go.

The hardest aspect of SLE and other chronic illnesses is there's no cure. However, you have books out there that state the cure is food. As for me, it goes dormant. You will always have one invader in you and if you eat something that triggers SLE it will wake up avenge with.

I hope that after reading this book, you will be able to know the symptoms and understand the frustration that it may put you through by my testimony and learn ways to be able to solve those problems. But again, remember to consult a naturopathic doctor. Your outcome will be much better than working with a traditional doctor. This book will be the first step into learning about your chronic illness. So many people who have this illness and don't know they have it or do not understand what to do. So many schools, doctors, nurses, teachers, and so many employers working for companies do not understand what lupus is. I hope you give this book to someone who may have lupus, someone who needs to understand what Lupus is. No one knows what the cause of this autoimmune disease. However, there is a lot of speculation that there could be a genetic link. I will never know due to all my family that would be genetically linked has passed away.

Here are some tips that I do to keep a positive day going outside of praying. I spread it out throughout the week and take it at night because that is when your body heals itself. Take a plant-based multivitamin, which is a preparation intended to serve as a dietary supplement with vitamins, minerals, and other nutritional elements. Calcium and magnesium are necessary for pH balance and protection against bone loss due to arthritis. I take L-cysteine 500 mg daily on an empty stomach. So, after dinner I wait an hour then take the L-cysteine. Take L-methionine with water or juice helps me get it down. I do not take it with milk it made me sick. I also take L-lysine with 50 mg, vitamin B6 and 100 mg vitamin C for better absorption. This assists in cellular protection and preservation. It is important in skin formation and my white blood cell activity. It also aids in preventing mouth sores and offers protection against viruses. Using proteolytic enzymes is for anti-inflammatory and antiviral agents I take it with a meal. I also place these in a smoothie with fruit and spinach and its good.

Taken essential fatty acids like black currant seed oil, flaxseed oil, ginger and primrose oil aid in my arthritis, protect my skin cells and are needed for the reproduction of all my body cells. Glucosamine sulfate and N-acetyl glucosamine is good for you. It helps with me having healthy connective tissue. It helps to prevent lupus erythematosus. Garlic is good to cook with if you do not want to take two capsules three times daily with meals. It is an immune system enhancer that protects enzyme systems. This was new to me. Raw thymus glandular, and raw spleen glandular did not work for me the smell alone made me think it was nasty. However, you may love it. Please use as directed on the label, but it is used to enhance the immune function. What is very important is getting with a naturopathic doctor and he/she will put you on a great health plan. You will see a big change!

My favorite that helps in the colds months is vitamin C with bioflavonoids. I take 1,000 to 2,000 mg daily this is based on my weight size. This aids in normalizing immune functions. I Take 50 to 100 mg of zinc, 3 mg of copper daily. I do not exceed the amount from the supplements that are provided. Copper aids in normalizing immune function, protects the skin and organs and promotes healing. The use of zinc gluconate lozenges or opt zinc for best absorption needs to balance with zinc. All the nutrients that I use are very important. My recommendations are a naturopathic doctor to provide your needs.

"That is why many among you are weak and sick, and a number of you have fallen asleep" (1 Corinthians 11:30). Listen to your body.

Listening will help you evaluate what could be going on while you are in remission.

As you read and do a lot of research, you will find that there are so many things that could be helpful for your body. I have tips of making myself feel better.

For example, acidophilus protects against intestinal bacterial imbalances. I use a nondairy formula and take it as directed on the label and on an empty stomach. Herpanacine from Diamond-Herpanacine Associates is also helpful. It contains a balance of antioxidants, amino acids, and herbs that promote my skin. Kelp and alfalfa supply commonly deficient minerals. Talk with your naturopathic doctor about taken what is noted above.

Taken mineral complex with vitamin B complex. For each major B vitamin, I take 50 mg three times daily with meals to supply commonly deficient nutrients. I use a high-quality hypoallergenic formula. This will help with healing mouth sores, protects against anemia, and protect the skin tissues. It is also important for brain function and digestion.

Cooking with Pycnogenol which is a grape seed extract that is a powerful antioxidant with free radical scavengers that protect the cells. Vitamin A with mixed carotenoids is a good supplement. Take natural beta-carotenoids 500 mg daily and carotenoid complex, better known as Betatene. The potent antioxidant and free radical scavenger are needed for tissue healing. It is an antioxidant and vitamin A precursor. Take B12 shots twice a month.

Last is vitamin E. This powerful antioxidant helps the body use oxygen more efficiently and promotes healing. There are many forms, but I find that D alpha tocopherol works for me. I know you are wondering how I take all this natural medication. I do it by putting it in a smoothie with fruit and vegetables, cooking with it or some of the food have it in them.

Here are some helpful herbs that I put in smoothies or cook with. Alfalfa is a good source of minerals needed for healing. Alcohol-free goldenseal extract is also good for inflammation. I place a few drops in my bath at bedtime or leave it on overnight for fast healing. I am allergic to ragweed, but for others, it may be beneficial in treating lupus, including burdock root, feverfew, and red clover. Try using licorice root as a tea or dilute it to alleviate lupus symptoms. If you are taking immunosuppressive agents such as steroids, you may find licorice root will provide comparable results without being as harmful to your system or causing you to gain weight. I do not take licorice because it elevates my blood pressure but again you check with your doctor.

The recommendation when eating is hard to explain because you have so much out there that is natural. Make sure to consult all your doctors and your bank account before trying the herbs or medications. This process is very expensive. You need to get your iron from food sources, not supplements. Taking iron in supplements contributes to pain, swelling, and joint destruction for me. I love eating Chinese food, but now I must avoid eating it because of the alfalfa sprouts. They contain Canavan, a toxic substance that is incorporated into protein in place of arginine. For some, you may need that but for me, that's a "no" I also get migraines. Get plenty of rest and regular moderate exercise that promotes muscle tone and fitness. Avoid strong sunlight and wear protection for the sun.

Protect your skin by applying a sunscreen product with an SPF of fifteen or higher. Wear a wide-brimmed hat and clothing that will cover exposed skin. Go out in the sun only when necessary.

I only use hypoallergenic soaps and cosmetics. Some deodorant soaps and other toiletry items may contain ingredients that will increase your sensitivity to light. Try to avoid fluorescent lighting in both the home and the workplace. Exposure to fluorescent lighting can aggravate lupus symptoms. If possible, remove all fluorescent and halogen lighting and replace it with incandescent bulbs. Avoid large groups of people and those with colds or other viral infections. I was told to avoid using birth control pills because they might cause my lupus to flare up. I never could get a good reason, so check with your doctor. When you have a flare-up, substances that are common contributing factors include chemicals, environmental pollutants, seasonings, and some foods. Have a test for food allergies done. It will be helpful to know what foods you need to stay away from.

However, many different treatments are used for lupus. Anti-inflammatory drugs are usually used first. Antimalarial drugs, such as hydroxychloroquine (Plaquenil), may alleviate the skin problems and sun sensitivity that afflict lupus.

In severe cases, physicians may have to use cortisone and immunosuppressive agents to induce remission. Corticosteroids, such as prednisone (Deltasone and others) are adrenal hormones that are considered important in the treatment of lupus.

Dehydroepiandrosterone (DHEA) therapy has been found to help in treating lupus. Radiation treatment for lupus, as I told about in my story, is in the experimental stages. It involves using low doses of radiation to the lymph nodes to suppress the immune system, and it did not work for me. I refused to use anticancer drugs to decrease both the immune system responsiveness and the need for steroids. Anti-cancer drugs may be toxic to the bone marrow and must be used with caution. Another experimental treatment for lupus involves plasmapheresis, a process in which harmful anti-antigen complexes are filtered out of the blood plasma. However, mild cases of lupus respond well to supplements that build up the immune system. Pray that you never have to come to this point.

When you are in pain from head to toe, Dermaka is an all-natural plant-based cream enriched with vitamins that can be used on all types of skin disorders secondary to anti-inflammatory, antimicrobial, and antioxidant properties. This is a great cream that I use, and you must use it twice a day to feel the difference. This product is clinically tested and has been shown to have a rapid resolution of inflammatory changes and bruising. This product is only available online. Let me not forget to add to get your eyes checked twice a year because some lupus medications can cause blindness.

> And on the banks, on both sides of the river, there will grow all kinds of trees for food. Their leaves will not wither, nor their fruit fails, but they will bear fresh fruit every month because the water for them flows from the sanctuary. Their fruit will be for food, and their leaves for healing. (Ezekiel 47:12)

God explains in 1 Corinthians 3:17 (ESV) that if anyone destroys God's temple, God will destroy him, for God's temple is holy, and you are that temple.

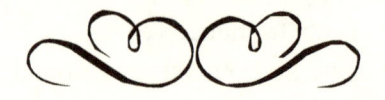

PEOPLE WILL NOT BELIEVE YOU/ME

I KNOW YOU are loving the information because it allows you to understand who I am and what I am going through. Most authors don't want you to know them. However, at this point, I am an open book. I now have over $50,000 in medical bills because nobody understands what lupus is about. It is good advice to continue to question your doctors until you get an understanding of their plan for your life. Don't allow them to do all the talking or make speculations because of the symptoms you tell them you are having at that moment. Pick yourself up. Don't become their test dummy.

For years, I prayed that someone would understand, and help me but not one person did. Everyone thought I was lying about my condition and my pain. I walk around looking stunning all the time and at one point one of my close family members told me to stop faking that I was only doing this for attention. People need to understand not to judge a book by its cover.

Judging a book by the cover makes me feel as if I am on this journey all alone. Why are my ears ringing? Why do my stomach and my body hurt, and why I am tired all the time? Lord, I am crying out to you. What is wrong? My job thought I just wanted time off work. I could not think straight when I am talking my voice sounds as if I am shaking from head to toe. I had to pause for a long period at times to remember what I was about to say. When I talked, my voice sounds as if I was nervous all the time, and my friends didn't think I wanted to spend time with them anymore. I cannot take this anymore.

Enough, enough, enough, damn, enough. I make the call; another doctor.

Walking around day by day, my smile had to be practiced for years so I would not show pain. I did not want people feeling sorry for me or saying, "How are you today?" They would not want the truth or had time for the truth. Even if I told them, all I get out of it is "I sorry you are going through" that or they become judgmental with questions. Maybe they may say I know someone that died from lupus. Every day, I must act as if everything is okay, but you would never, ever know that internally because I feel awful. I feel like I walk around as if I have the flu.

Going to church, I always thank the Lord blessing me with another day, for waking me up in the morning. Still, I found myself not at peace. So, I prayed, "Heavenly Father, please place your hands on me right now." As I continued with prayer., I can hear "Don't give up. I have more for you to do."

Never could I understand, but there was something inside of me that made me realize that I needed to continue to find out more about my health condition, to give my time back to the less fortunate, and to be an advocate for this cause by spreading the word about my issue. I need to let people know what I'm going through. I am just a vessel that God is allowing me to do his work. He is not done with me yet so obey and accept the things that you cannot change and have the wisdom to know the difference.

As you continue to read, you will learn that lupus does not take a day off. Every day is full of stiffness, pain, keeping the blinds closed, having a slow start when you wake up and lots of pain. At some points in my life I would feel lost. When I wake up, life would tell me that I am not forgotten, so listen to your lupus when it's talking to you."

> "If you are ever alone, this is a time to rethink your approach to life; You cannot replace the connection you had in the past but little by little you can rebuild again."

—LaTonya Bias, Phd

POEM

I hope you have a rock in your life that will stand out for you as you read this poem. When you are reading, say your rock's name at the end of each question.

You Are My Rock

Who has been by my side other than God?
Who has prayed harder than any pastor in the United States?
Who made me strong with wisdom?
Who is my best friend?
Who are the best moms, dads, sisters, aunts, and uncles in the world?
Who is there when my times are hard no matter if he/she is in pain?
Who helps me through my issues when they have their own?
Who loves unconditionally?
Who is my ride or die?
Who fights for my rights?
Who tells me that I am wrong?
Who works endlessly to help people and their communities?
Who let the sunshine in when all I wanted was the blinds to be closed?
Who taught me about how to budget?
Who reintroduced me to God?
I could go on and on, but you know you are, "my rock". You are my rock, rock, rock, rock, rock.
Love you!

It is time for you to act, O Lord your law is being broken.
(Psalm 119:126 NIV)

NEXT STEPS

ACTS TAKING THE next steps in your life. This will help you defend and avoid judgment and disappointments. When you wake up, thank the Lord that you woke up. You are not guaranteed tomorrow, so make the best out of your day. You are not going to feel like moving, but what I do is first start out by stretching. I have set my alarm two hours before I get my day started. Start with your hands. Wiggle each finger back and forth until you can feel the blood flowing through them. Next, move your wrist and then your full arm. Invest in a soft rubber ball to us on the bottom of your feet. As you sit on the side of the bed, place your feet on top of the ball and roll your feet back and forth until you can feel the blood flowing through them. This will get the blood circulating through your body.

Try doing neck rotations and lateral neck flexion when you wake up and have your legs hanging off the side of the bed. Next, turn your head slowly to look over one shoulder, then the other shoulder. Hold your head in each direction for five seconds. Repeat this process ten times, and do it twice a day, once in the day and once at night before you go to bed.

Slowly tilt your head toward one shoulder, and then tilt your head to the other shoulder and hold for five seconds. Repeat these ten times two times a day. This will help with your cervical spine. Don't forget to bend your head forward and backward and hold for five seconds and repeat these ten times two times a day. Doing this allows you to loosen up your body to get you through the day.

Now you can start with your legs, stand up. Move them from side to side. Then attempt to pull your body down to touch the floor. Now do not move just yet. You want to pay attention to your body and allow all the blood to flow in its proper places. Stand back up and move your legs again from side to side. If you do not feel light-headed, bend down and touch your toes again. You should feel like moving around after this. This helps me every day. Last, sit down on the edge of the bed and drink a bottle of water.

The reason I say bottle because you would need to keep water by your bed throughout the night. The water cannot be in an open bottle because it will build up dust and bacterial on the top surface of your open container. So please keep a closed bottle or cover your cup with a napkin.

> "Trust in the Lord with all your heart and lean not on your understanding, in all your ways acknowledge him, and he shall direct your paths.
>
> Proverbs 3:5-6

WHAT CAN I EAT?

MIGRAINES CAN COME in many forms, but I must avoid the following:

- Monosodium glutamate (Chinese Food here- MSG is found in BBQ, Korean, Ramen, Japanese, and even popular spice mixtures like Lowry's and Everglades)
- Onions
- Vinegar (except white vinegar)
- Peanut butter
- Nuts, especially peanuts
- Pizza
- Avocadoes
- Fermented sausage (salami, pepperoni, bologna, hotdogs)
- Anything fermented, pickled, or marinated
- Chicken livers
- Sour cream
- Hot, fresh bread, doughnuts
- Canned figs
- Herring
- Chocolate
- Yogurt
- Pods or broad beans (lima, navy, and peapods)
- Excessive tea or coffee, pop/cola
- Excessive citrus foods
- Excessive pork
- Excessive bananas

- Ripened cheese (cheddar, brie, stilton, gruyere, cemental, camembert)
- Alcoholic beverages, especially champagne, beer, red wines, bourbon, gin, and vodka

I know you are thinking, *Well, what I can eat*. Remember, those foods are to avoid migraines. Those are just a few triggers and remember that those are what I have found affect me and were recommended by my doctors not to take. There are times when a change in the weather can become a trigger. Sleep deprivation and poor sleep habits can also lead to headaches, especially migraine attacks. Though hypoglycemia is a rare cause of headaches, eating three meals at regular intervals and small quantities is important in helping control migraines. The stress of school or exams may precipitate headaches. These stresses cannot be avoided, but with appropriate relaxation techniques, they can be minimized. For example, get a massage twice a month. Breathe in through your nose and out your mouth for a few minutes.

Here are more triggers that I cannot ignore:

- Perfume
- Gasoline
- Various food odors
- An excess number of extracurricular activities
- Relationships with friends, siblings, or parents
- Disruption of lifestyle
- Feeling bummed out

All those points noted above are life. Make sure that you are at 75% healthy when taken on these triggers.

CELEBRITIES WITH LUPUS

YOU FIND THAT a lot of people do not talk about their autoimmune systems. There are a few celebrities who are open about lupus and only talk about it when asked.

- Selena Gomez
- Nick Cannon
- Lady Gaga
- Toni Braxton
- Seal
- Cori Broadus (Snoop Doggy's daughter)
- Tim Raines (baseball player, 1999)
- Charles Kuralt (journalist, died)
- Flannery O'Connor (novelist, died)
- Michael Wayne (son of John Wayne)
- Lauren Shuler Donner (producer, *X-Men*)

All these names are public information, so you should look them up and read more about their stories.

> Jesus went throughout Galilee teaching in their synagogues preaching the good news of the kingdom and healing every disease and sickness among the people. (Matthew 4:23, 10:1)

Find a church home that can pray for you and get into a life group or Bible study. The disciples come when getting closer to God. Pray the evil spirits away, and for healing over this disease.

RECOMMENDATION

IF YOU STILL want to go, see a doctor after all this information you just read. When going to the doctor, make sure you have a guide with questions. You live with lupus every day, but you probably see your rheumatologist only once every three months or so. Most appointments last less than fifteen minutes, and you are sitting most of the time, so it's important to make the most of the valuable time you spend with your doctors. I am going to provide you with some steps to follow that are designed to help you have the power to "face your lupus". This will allow you to make your time productive.

Take note of all your symptoms, even the ones that may not feel like lupus. Make sure that you monitor and track your symptoms daily. Document how lupus is affecting your life. Explain how it is interfering with your day-to-day functions. This will allow you to see a pattern over time and become prepared the next time it comes around. Make sure you put the starting points on the calendar of any issue that occurs. Talk to someone you trust and to be your support system when you have fogs. That way if you forget something your support will be there for you. Have all your other doctors' or specialists' medical records and current medications sent to each other so that all doctors will be on the same page. Be ready to answer some common physician questions. The ones I receive the most are, "How have you been feeling physically? How have you been feeling emotionally? Anything significant in your life I should know about? Any new problems I should be aware of?" If your doctor does not ask you these questions or close to these questions, find a new doctor.

I have done other treatments that I found very effective, but please consult your doctor before using these things. One is Bio freeze. Bio freeze manages pain and allows you to take part in the activities you enjoy the most like moving. When I am resting at night and receive pain in my leg or back. I roll over and put the Bio freeze on. Chiropractors, who I recommend that you see monthly, state that the Bio freeze is the number-one clinically used and recommended topical pain reliever among them, physical therapists, massage therapists, and podiatrists all use Bio freeze. I am not getting paid to tell you about this product. However, this is great to use. Bio freeze provides penetrating, long-lasting pain relief for arthritis, sore muscles joints, and back pain. Try putting it on in the morning or at night. The time-tested, paraben-free formula uses soothing menthol as the active ingredient and features other herbal ingredients. I use this product as needed, and it is a lifesaver.

Not sure if you all heard about Traumeel. When I was seeing my chiropractor, he told me about Traumeel. He explained that it is a pain reliever and inflammation without the risk of steroids. Traumeel is a combination of twelve plant medicines and two mineral extracts. All fourteen of these medicines are micro-dosed and are intended to stimulate your body to resolve its pain. Remember, these are my recommendation and I am not a doctor, so talk with your doctor about using Traumeel. I have not had any issues with the product.

You may know about Myers' Cocktail. If this is your first time, then please talk with your doctor because this had not been evaluated by the Food and Drug Administration. None of the medications or recommendations are intended to diagnose, treat, cure, or prevent any disease. This is my journey, and these things have worked for me. The Myers' Cocktail is an intramuscular vitamin injection that works by increasing the blood concentration of several essential vitamins and minerals beyond that which can be achieved when injected. The Myers' Cocktail is named for the late John Myers, MD, a Maryland physician who used injections of nutrients to treat many chronic conditions.

The ingredients in the Myers' Cocktail are vitamin C, multiple B vitamins (B1, B2, B3, B5, B6, and B12) magnesium, taurine, zinc, selenium, copper, chromium, potassium, and molybdenum. The Myers' Cocktail help treat fatigue, upper respiratory tract infections, chronic sinusitis, seasonal allergic rhinitis, asthma, migraines, musculoskeletal disorders, fibromyalgia, and other disorders. It is not a cure it just helps. There are adverse effects, like soreness at the site of injection twenty-four to forty-eight hours after administration. There might be a strong urine odor six to eight hours after injection, siting, increased heart rate, and increased energy levels. You can have an allergic reaction if you are sensitive to one or more ingredients I stated. Make sure you talk with your doctor and disclose all medications or medical conditions before receiving the injection. I get an injection during the winter months or allergy season. My insurance does not cover the injections, but I find it is worth it.

EXERCISE DAILY

WHEN IT COMES to exercise, I do a light workout daily. The reason is some of the foods make you gain weight fast. Doing light exercise is good. My lower back hurts because I sit most of the day when working. For the lower back, I do trunk rotation stretches. Keeping my back flat and feet together, I rotate my knees from side to side. I then hold for five seconds and repeat ten times on each side and do these two times per day. Next, try working on your pelvis. I find pelvic tilts are also good. This helps me keep a flat stomach. Flatten your back by tightening your stomach muscles and buttocks and hold for five seconds and repeat ten times two times a day. Over time you will see a change. However, make sure you do a "knee-to-chest stretch" by putting one hand behind one knee. Pull your knee into your chest until you feel a comfortable stretch in your lower back and buttocks. That helps me get off the floor after all the stomach work. Make sure you keep your back relaxed and hold for five seconds and repeat with the other knee ten times two times a day. I do this before I get out of bed and when I work out.

Lupus is a complicated, unpredictable disease whose symptoms can vary from person to person. Sometimes, though, it can be hard to remember all your symptoms, especially if are in remission. Make sure that you share your information with all the naturopathic doctors, eat right, and do light exercises daily, and that will help you have a healthier life.

CLASSIFICATIONS TO UNDERSTAND

I WANT TO explain to you some classifications of words and provide some examples for people to help them understand what I am saying.

Exercise is like muscle. Bone is living tissue that responds to exercise by becoming stronger. The best activity for your bones is weight-bearing exercises that force you to work against gravity. Remember that with weight-bearing exercises, less weight with more repetitions will go a long way. Some examples include walking, climbing stairs, lightweight training, and slow dancing. Exercising is challenging for me and others with lupus who are affected by joint pain and inflammation, muscle pain, and fatigue. However, I regularly exercise, and it helps prevent bone loss and provides many other health benefits.

HAIR LOSS

Maybe you've been losing your hair, wondering if this is normal. Why would this disease lead to hair loss? And is there anything that can be done? This is a great chapter to read if you enjoy your hair. I have a short and savvy hairstyle. My hair has always been thin. It would only grow to my shoulders. As I got older, I found myself wanting to keep it short, not because I liked the hairstyles, but because my hair was becoming thinner. I decided to do some research to see if lupus or the medication that I was taking could cause hair loss. Well, I got my answer and unfortunately it was yes. Lupus causes widespread inflammation that usually involves your skin, particularly on your face and scalp. Lupus can cause the hair on your scalp to gradually thin out, although a few people lose clumps of hair. Loss of eyebrows, eyelashes, and body hair are also possible. Thinking about it now, for some places where gray was growing, I was happy to lose that hair. Lol!

In most cases, your hair may grow back but slowly and only if the hair follicle did not come from the root. However, some people with lupus develop round (discoid) lesions on the scalp and only see a few or no fine strands of hair in the discoid part. Because these discoid lesions scar your hair follicles, they do cause permanent hair loss. As for me, my discoid is on both my front temporal lobes.

Lupus can also cause the scalp hair along your hairline to become fragile and break off easily, leaving you with a thin hairline appearance known as baby hair. Some people will use a toothbrush—yes, a real toothbrush—with styling gel to hold down what little hair they have on the hairline. Hair loss may be an early sign of lupus before the disease is diagnosed. But many other disorders can cause hair loss, so consult with your doctor if you notice unusual hair thinning or hair loss.

Women love hair color but do not think about the chemicals that may contribute to your hair loss because of your autoimmune disease. Lupus and the loss of hair can be devastating. Unfortunately, this means that it can potentially destroy our hair follicles, and some lupus patients begin losing patches of hair, leading to alopecia (bald spots).

Systemic lupus tends to cause flare-ups. In other words, there are times when the symptoms are worse than others. During these flares, hair loss can be intense. The good news is that hair often grows back once treatment is received, although it can be up to six months before things seem back to normal. If your hair loss is caused by the lupus medication (or other medication), the hair will usually grow back when the medication is out of your system, which could take a year.

If you want to prevent hair loss, one thing I recommend is to seek immediate advice from a naturopathic doctor. Early treatment can help alter your dosage or change your medication if it seems that the medication is causing your hair loss. I will color my hair black, thinking it would make me look younger. Plus, I wanted my gray to be covered. Well, someone very special who is a hairstylist told me that the black color was too harsh on my face. The black made me look older. She recommended going lighter. I took her advice, and it does bring joy to my life knowing people think that I am younger. Putting color in your hair may cause flare-ups of systemic lupus. Keep a diary and keep tabs on when having triggers. You can also do the following:

- Keep a low-stress level.
- Avoid the sun.
- Get enough rest.
- Avoid halogen or fluorescent lights.
- Act fast when you feel any infections coming on.
- Don't assume hair loss is associated with lupus.
- Keep your hair clean. (once or twice a week)

As I mentioned, lupus or systemic lupus erythematosus is a condition marked by a wide range of symptoms. Alopecia, the medical term for hair loss, affects roughly 45 percent of people with lupus. With lupus, there are generally two forms of hair loss. One is related to discoid lupus and results in scarring. The other is non-scarring. Scarring alopecia most commonly results from lupus associated with skin diseases alone, such as discoid lupus erythematosus or subacute cutaneous lupus rather than with systemic (all-over) lupus. In these conditions, lupus interferes with the normal function of the hair follicle. With systemic lupus, hair loss can be either diffuse (all over) or localized. When it is localized, it occurs most commonly on the front part of the scalp.

It's not unusual to shampoo with natural products (go to lovelifelupusfoundation.org to get the best shampoo, conditioner and leave-in) or comb your hair and find several stray hairs in the sink or shower. Sometimes it may even seem like more than normal. But losing fifty to a hundred hairs a day is perfectly common. I use a large, wide-tooth comb when my hair is wet so I will get very little breakage. I go to the salon once a week, and I have my hairstylist use a large, wide-tooth comb when she is doing my hair. She makes sure that the hair is placed correctly inside to curling irons so that he/she will not cause more breakage. However, 90 percent of a person's hair is growing at any given moment, with the remaining 10 percent in a resting phase. Your hair feeds off your bloodstream so the growth phase, anagen, can last from two to six years, after which the hair follicle enters the resting phase, telogen, which lasts about three months. After the resting phase, the hair is shed. New hair grows where the last one shed, and the cycle begins again. So, if you hear your hairstylist tell you that they have the hands to grow hair, you know that is a lie because you know the facts now.

There are many reasons why a person might experience hair loss in addition to those caused by lupus. Those reasons include the following:

- Heredity/genetics: Known medically as androgenetic alopecia, hereditary hair loss and thinning is the most common cause of hair loss. Typically, women will experience thinning hair while there is no cure for this form of hair loss, but natural supplements may help stem the onset.
- Alopecia aerate: A bit of a mystery, alopecia aerate is believed to be an autoimmune disease in which the body forms antibodies that attack its hair. The disease causes hair loss marked by totally smooth, round patches about the size of a coin or larger. It may even result in complete loss of scalp and body hair, though this is rare.
- Chemical treatments: Hair dyes, tints, bleaches, straighteners, relaxers, perms, combing with small combs when wet, and other hair products with chemicals can cause weakness of the hair, making it brittle and causing it to break and fall out. If you encounter this form of alopecia, simply stop using chemicals and talk with a naturopathic doctor.
- Telogen effluvium: Many people lose hair after a severe illness or surgery when anesthesia was used, as a result of stress, as well as after pregnancy. Those are the most common, but there could be more.
- Tinea: Fungal infections can lead to hair loss.
- Traumatic alopecia: Continuously playing with hair can cause hair breakage.
- Thyroid conditions: Both hypo and hyperthyroidism can lead to hair loss.
- Nutritional deficiencies: Deficiencies in protein, iron, biotin, zinc, and vitamin D are all associated with hair loss.

For me, it was very important to get a diagnosis for the loss of my hair. Making the correct diagnosis about the causes of your hair loss is important. If your hair loss is related to a flare-up of a disease (telogen effluvium), it will regrow in time. Non-lupus causes, ranging from fungal infections to thyroid disorders, need to be ruled out, rather than simply assuming the hair loss is due to your lupus. Your naturopathic doctor needs to know, and that way he or she can recognize your symptoms and diagnose you based on your history, physical exam, and laboratory tests. Sometimes a skin biopsy of the scalp may need to be done to determine the reasons.

I wanted to know if my hair loss was permanent. Well, yes and no. I read, depending on what you are doing with your body and hair. Many people worry that their hair loss with lupus will be permanent, and it can be at times. Whether your hair will return depends on the cause of the loss. As stated, there are several different reasons why this can occur. Doctors say that hair loss with lupus is reversible once treatment begins. As for me, when I received treatment, my hair came back as fuzz. When hair loss occurs due to scarring involving the hair follicle, the loss may be permanent. Discoid lupus is a major cause of scarring alopecia.

My naturopathic doctor said that the best way to treat hair loss caused by lupus is to treat the underlying disease by getting it under control. Besides, when your disease is controlled, some of the natural plant supplements can be taken not as often for the improvement in your hair loss. People have tried several nutritional supplements, for example, biotin, but some dietary supplements and water (spring, distilled) may interfere with some medications or natural plant-based supplements. It is important to talk to your naturopathic doctor before taking any supplements.

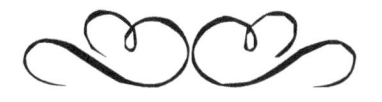

COPING

I HAVE HAD lupus for a long time and coping with lupus is frustrating not only for me but also for my family. While many of the other symptoms of lupus are more concerning from a medical standpoint, the butterfly on my face is something that you can see each time you look at me or I look in the mirror. That is why I found it was very important to talk to my naturopathic doctor about any issues I have with my lupus. Since I have had lupus, sometimes a good makeup artist can minimize the appearance of the spots on my face. I have not found a company that can cover my spots without having hard chemicals in the products. Overall, dealing with a chronic disease like lupus can be challenging. Concerns about your health and the effects of lupus on your work and family life can be stressful. Talk to your naturopathic doctor and others about your symptoms and feelings. You also may want to consider counseling or joining a support group (lovelifelupusfoundation.org). Many people find it helpful to talk to others who may be having similar experiences.

I heard this word *remission* from one of my old doctors. I wanted to know what that meant. Remission is a decrease in or disappearance of signs and symptoms. In partial remission, some, but not all, signs and symptoms have disappeared, although they still may be in your body.

However, everyone who lives with lupus will experience the disease differently. The symptoms vary, and not all people will suffer from the same ones. Remission is the time when lupus isn't active. It also varies greatly from person to person. Some lupus patients will suffer from mild symptoms constantly (flare-ups) without any remission; others may have more severe symptoms but have periods of remission.

The frequency of flares and remission depends on the person, but according to a lupus foundation, the first five years of lupus tend to be the most uncertain, for the patient and the rheumatologist. This can make treating lupus quite challenging during those initial years. There are steps lupus patients can take to help stay in remission. These include taking the supplements the naturopathic doctor prescribes, not overdoing things daily, avoiding stress as much as possible, eating well, getting plenty of quality sleep so your body can heal, light exercising, maintaining healthy body weight, and avoiding UV rays. Looking after yourself physically and emotionally will help keep flares at low and keep you in remission longer, helping you enjoy a fulfilling life with lupus.

SUPPORT SYSTEM

WHEN DEALING WITH one of my diagnoses, I struggled to recover from atrial fibrillation and adjust to the debilitating effects of joint and muscle inflammation and pain. Atrial fibrillation, or AFib, is a quivery, fluttery heartbeat. You might also hear the doctor call its arrhythmia. It means your heart's normal rhythm is out of whack. Because your blood isn't moving well, you're more likely to have heart failure. That's when your heart can't keep up with your body's needs. Blood can also pool inside your heart and form clots. If one gets stuck in your brain, you can have a stroke. I felt like the aspirations I had for my life had been cast out beyond my reach. How could I achieve my dreams? What would happen to my children? I need to find a funeral home; I must save money for my children because I want to break the chain of brokenness in my family. When I could hardly lift my arms high enough to undress, I always had thoughts about death coming soon.

A support system is important for a patient who is afflicted with any lifelong disease. Having someone you can frequently lean on for emotional support can keep your life-forces up. Identify key people in your life who can be a constant source of support, whether it's your family members, coworkers, or close friends. Additionally, the naturopathic doctor and support groups you've been meeting with regularly can also serve as support. They're more knowledgeable about your disease than others due to their expertise, so be sure to connect with them. In a support group, you can befriend those who are going through the same issues as you. You may find that communicating with them is awkward or difficult at first but rest assured that they will be there to help and most importantly, listen.

Once you have selected the right people, inform them that you've chosen them to be your support group. They are very helpful in the event of an emergency since they can accompany you to the hospital and communicate with any medical personnel for any special requests.

My friends existed in a world I could not function in the bustling, vigorous existence of working, studying, taking care of a home, and being a wife into the early-morning hours. My life has been snatched, replaced by swallowing pills and being pain riddled. I watched the life I thought I would be living and the worried expressions of my friends and family drift farther and farther away. No matter how much I told my family and friends I didn't feel good, I cannot do your hair, the understanding of my health condition did not click since I was able to smile, walk, talk, and dance, which I love to do left me isolated.

I felt isolated for years. When speaking to family and friends, I would get questions I did not know how to answer. I became lost, longing for the sense of belonging I used to have with so-called normal, healthy society, but all this changed.

The key is to avoid isolation, as it can drag you down. Connecting with a support group can provide a sense of reaffirmation that you're not alone in your struggle. Learning from their stories is a way to create a deeper bond with them. Become a part of a church group. You will find that some churches have the same beliefs you do and will take you in like you have been a part of their lives for a long time. You can learn a lot from people who have had lupus longer than you. Due to their experience, they can provide pointers on what to watch out for and other techniques that can help you cope with lupus easier. In time, you can provide help to newly joined members, and they can look up to you, creating a positive atmosphere of support, hope, and friendship.

In the end, it's entirely possible to enjoy life with lupus. All it takes is a determination on your part (proper nutrition and exercise) to better manage the symptoms, the help of a strong support group, and alternative treatment methods for lupus. Alternative treatments for lupus typically seek to manage symptoms rather than to cure the disease. Many herbal supplements advertised as providing relief for lupus symptoms are untested and unproven. There is a new one called Turmeric CBD. They may have limited effectiveness, and they could interact with other treatments and supplements to cause even greater problems because it is not FDA approved.

SUPPLEMENT

SOME LUPUS PATIENTS find that when they take supplements containing dehydroepiandrosterone, commonly known as DHEA, they're able to cut back on the steroids controlling their symptoms. When I define steroids, the first thing that comes to mind is the word *fat*. No matter what, when I take steroids, I blow up like OVER two hundred pounds. Steroids are a large group of chemical substances classified by a specific carbon structure. Steroids include drugs used to relieve swelling and inflammation, such as prednisone cortisone; and vitamin D. Prednisone is a synthetic corticosteroid that mimics the action of cortisol (hydrocortisone), the naturally occurring corticosteroid produced in the body by the adrenal glands.

Corticosteroids have many effects on the body, but they most often are used for their potent anti-inflammatory effects, particularly in those diseases and conditions in which the immune system plays an important role, for example, arthritis, colitis, asthma, bronchitis, skin problems, and allergies, to name a few.

I hate omega-3s. My stomach hurts every time I take them. However, the omega-3 fatty acids in fish oil supplements also show potential in treating lupus, as does vitamin D. Primrose oil, S-adenosylmethionine, and flaxseed oil may also have anti-inflammatory properties that help relieve lupus symptoms. However, some herbal supplements can make lupus symptoms worse. For instance, lupus patients who have overactive immune systems already should avoid taking echinacea, an herbal supplement that provides an unneeded boost to the immune system. Because of the danger of creating new problems, a lupus patient should only begin treatment with supplements after discussing her case with her doctor. Besides some supplements may interfere with the proper working of prescribed supplements from a naturopathic doctor.

PAIN

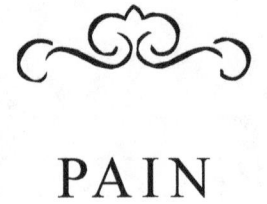

IN MY EXPERIENCE with pain, there is no reliever out there to help. If you take medication, it only temporarily subsides the pain. However, the pain will wake you up out of your sleep. Most doctors recommend a traditional course of nonsteroidal, anti-inflammatory drugs, such as ibuprofen or aspirin, to treat the inflammation and pain of lupus. However, because these drugs can have unwanted side effects, lupus patients often turn to alternative methods of pain control, such as acupuncture, which shows some signs of efficacy in treating lupus pain. I never tried acupuncture because my skin is too sensitive, so trying acupuncture will not work for me. Many chat groups, friends have said that it works for them.

Meditation help me deal with my pain and have some control management. Also, the time-tested pain relief methods of hot and cold compresses can provide immediate pain relief for me. My number one key, and I wish that my insurance company had this as a part of my plan, is having massages. A massage by a licensed massage therapist can help ease the swelling and joint pain that is associated with lupus. If you have a version of lupus that affects the skin, however, you should avoid massage therapy, as it can cause severe bruising. If not, getting up from the table after a rub from head to toe for an hour or two will put you on the right path for the week. Seeing the chiropractor four times out of the month helps me keep everything in place. I found that chiropractors can see where you are inflamed and advise you what to do on treating those areas.

It still goes through my mind that lupus is an autoimmune disease that has no cure. While traditional medicines can try to control lupus, they do not always provide complete relief from the pain and joint swelling that the disease often causes. While some alternative treatment methods for lupus are unproven and others may even be dangerous, there are several options for lupus patients seeking some unconventional relief.

If you're looking for new approaches to add to your lupus pain management toolkit, you might want to consider a few treatments outside of conventional, or mainstream, medicine. Some of the methods might stray just off the path of conventional medicine and into complementary and alternative medicine (CAM). CAM is defined as a group of diverse medical and healthcare systems, practices, and products that are not presently considered to be part of conventional, Western medicine. You might also see CAM referred to as "complementary and integrative health," which is a newer term for the same idea.

It is important to note at the beginning current lupus foundations will not recommend medications, products, or methods that are not approved by the Food and Drug Administration (FDA) or the American College of Rheumatology. One reason people do not understand because you have groups and bloggers stating, "remedies that have not undergone the scrutiny of scientific investigation, lack the crucial information and data necessary to enable physicians to make sound recommendations regarding substances." Therefore, after reading that statement, it is important to understand your concerns and do lots of research with credible sites. As for me, I will spread the word and help find a cure until the day I die.

Here's an introduction to four complementary and alternative medicine (CAM) methods that are sometimes used for lupus pain management. These approaches are innovative to some and completely familiar to others. The methods themselves have been in use by various cultures for thousands of years.

Meditation is a conscious mental process using certain techniques, such as focusing your attention or maintaining a specific posture, to relax your body and mind by suspending your stream of consciousness thoughts. For health purposes, use it to increase physical relaxation, mental calmness, and psychological balance or to cope with one or more diseases and conditions and for overall wellness. For with me and lupus, meditation may help to ease pain, depression, and stress. The biggest benefit may be overall wellness. Scientists aren't sure yet how meditation affects the body specifically or what specific influence it has on overall health. It's generally a safe technique, although some studies have suggested that intensive meditation may worsen symptoms.

Many people with chronic pain issues like lupus explore massage therapy. Like myself, twice a month is mandatory. Massage therapy, as a practice, dates back thousands of years. There are many types of massage, including pressing, rubbing, and moving muscles and other soft tissues of the body, primarily by using the hands and fingers. The treatments often last for thirty minutes to an hour and can be performed in an office. As for me, I need two hours.

The goal of massage therapy is to increase blood flow and oxygen to the area being massaged. You may find that this reduces swelling, alleviates pain, promotes relaxation, and reduces stress. However, I must drink lots of water after having a massage because my lips look like I have created a new lipstick called "flour". Again, if you're considering massage therapy, first talk to your healthcare provider, and then, if you proceed, find a licensed massage therapist.

I love music that tells a story. Music is a big part of my life. I remember my mom turning on music to clean our house. I would see my family when we would have gatherings listening to music and dancing reflecting joy in their lives. For me, relaxing music can also reduce stress. At times, I could not find a good pain management treatment. I have been to doctors to help control the pain, and I ended up with over six prescriptions. The best treatment for systemic lupus erythematosus depends on the patient and her healthcare practitioner. You might explore different ways to manage your lupus pain throughout your life. As you consider different approaches, including complementary and integrative health, remember that people react differently to treatment plans and while a method that works for me may not work at all for you.

None of these treatments should replace your regular medical care or delay you seeing a naturopathic doctor about any problems. These treatments may help relieve your symptoms, but they don't affect survival rates or remissions. Help me find a cure. Spread the word and bring awareness about Lupus. Tell them what you have learned about this book and go onto the website Lovelifelupusfoundation.org to learn more.

YOU ARE VERY SICK

IN 2000, I saw a new rheumatologist, and the truth struck me hard in the face. I had high levels for my kidneys, and they wanted to watch me weekly so I would not get too severe. I remember when she told me. She held my hands, looked in my eyes, and said, "I am sorry. You have to get on disability." Well, my salon career was over, and life would never be the same. I could not cook, clean, or do fun things outside with my children. The bed became my life. I must admit that I was angry with myself. I kept thinking that if I had taken it seriously from the beginning, perhaps it could have been controlled.

Perhaps it wouldn't have advanced to this level of severity. I realized the denial I had been in, and I knew that something had to change. Just as losing a loved one can cause a downward spiral of emotional turmoil, so can the discovery of a chronic illness. Gaining lupus acceptance does not just happen. It is a process that must be knowledgeable.

Oftentimes the emotional reaction to the illness can be more restricting than the illness itself, and it is only through the adjustment process that I can truly embrace the new person I have become. Regardless of the severity, lupus will change you. The illness establishes itself in several physical and emotional challenges (like having to deal with lupus, stress, and depression). I discovered limitations that I never expected. My energy levels and well-being declined, medications become a priority, and doctors' appointments seemed never-ending. I must remind the doctors all the time when they are prescribing another prescription to check and make sure that it does not have a reaction from other medications I am taking. Clearly, changing my mindset was essential, working on that will change my process of thinking.

You only get one life, so I don't want to be known for one thing but for everything I do.

—LaTonya Bias

FIBROMYALGIA AND OSTEOPOROSIS

I THINK IT is important that you know what fibromyalgia is about. Fibromyalgia is a disorder characterized by widespread musculoskeletal pain accompanied by fatigue, sleep, memory and mood issues. Researchers believe that fibromyalgia amplifies painful sensations by affecting the way your brain processes pain signals. Some doctors will diagnose you with fibromyalgia because your lupus test results do not show you have lupus. According to the National Institutes of Health (NIH), there is a link between lupus and fibromyalgia and osteoporosis.

What is osteoporosis? Osteoporosis is a condition in which the bones become less dense and more likely to fracture. Fractures from osteoporosis can result in significant pain and disability. In the United States, more than 53 million people either already have osteoporosis or are at high risk due to low bone mass.

Risk factors for developing osteoporosis include the following:

- thinness or small frame
- family history of the disease
- being postmenopausal and particularly having had an early menopause
- abnormal absence of menstrual periods (amenorrhea)
- prolonged use of certain medications, such as those used to treat lupus, asthma, thyroid deficiencies, and seizures
- low calcium intake
- lack of physical activity
- smoking
- excessive alcohol intake

The doctors say that osteoporosis often can be prevented. It is known as a silent disease because, if undetected, bone loss can progress for many years without symptoms until a fracture occurs. Osteoporosis has been called a childhood disease with old-age consequences because building healthy bones in youth helps prevent osteoporosis and fractures later in life. However, it is never too late to adopt new habits for a healthy life. I found that there are links between lupus and osteoporosis.

Studies have found an increase in bone loss and fracture in individuals with SLE. Individuals with lupus are at increased risk for osteoporosis for many reasons. I have found that not one doctor has recommended to treat me for osteoporosis even though my lower back has started to have bone loss. I have read up on how to treat bone loss. I would begin with the glucocorticoid medications often prescribed to treat SLE, which can trigger significant bone loss. In addition, pain and fatigue caused by the disease can result in inactivity, further increasing osteoporosis risk. Studies also show that bone loss in lupus may occur as a direct result of the disease. The fact that 90 percent of the people affected with lupus are women, a group already at increased risk for osteoporosis. Also, management strategies for the prevention and treatment of osteoporosis in people with lupus are not significantly different from the strategies for those who do not have the disease.

It is very important to focus on nutrition. You want to have a well-balanced diet that is rich in calcium and vitamin D. This is important for healthy bones. Good sources of calcium include low-fat dairy products, not excluding dark green, leafy vegetables and calcium-fortified foods and purified drinking water. Supplements can help ensure that you get adequate amounts of calcium each day, especially in people with a proven milk allergy.

The Institute of Medicine recommends a daily calcium intake of 1,000 mg for women up to age fifty. Women over age fifty should increase their intake to 1,200 mg daily. I drink very little milk, so I take supplements for support. I also must admit, I am bad at having a well-balanced diet. I try to have fruits and vegetables in a smoothie in the morning, a small meal in the afternoon, and a balanced meal for dinner. I eat no meat, rice, potatoes, and pasta because I have high blood pressure. This goes against the world's ways of eating. If you want to take control of your body, pay attention to what you put in it.

My naturopathic doctor prescribes me vitamin D. Vitamin D plays an important role in calcium absorption and bone health. Food sources of vitamin D include egg yolks, saltwater fish, and liver. I cannot benefit from them because I do not eat it. Many people obtain enough vitamin D naturally, but some individuals may need vitamin D supplements to achieve the recommended intake of 600 to 800 mg each day.

LIFESTYLE

MY LIFESTYLE IS laid back, no getting mad, I talk things through, and I try to stay away from people that smoke because second hand is real. Smoking is bad for your bones as well as the heart and lungs. Women who smoke tend to go through menopause earlier, resulting in earlier reduction in levels of the bone-preserving hormone estrogen and triggering earlier bone loss. Also, smokers may absorb less calcium from their diets. Alcohol also can have a negative effect on bone health. Those who drink heavily are more prone to bone loss because of poor nutrition and an increased risk of falling. I know it may feel like you cannot do anything. However, if you want to live to see your destiny fulfilled, then don't drink or smoke.

I recommend a bone density test every five years. A bone mineral density (BMD) test measures bone density at various parts of the body. This safe and painless test can detect osteoporosis before a fracture occurs and predict one's chances of fracturing in the future. Lupus patients, particularly those receiving glucocorticoid therapy for two months or more, should talk to their doctors about whether they might be candidates for a BMD test. The BMD test can help determine whether medication should be considered.

Like lupus, osteoporosis is a disease with no cure. However, several supplements are available for the prevention and/or treatment. Studies have found an increased risk of bone loss and fracture in individuals with rheumatoid arthritis. People with rheumatoid arthritis are at increased risk for osteoporosis for many reasons. To begin with, glucocorticoid medications, which are often prescribed for the treatment of rheumatoid arthritis, can trigger significant bone loss. Besides, pain and loss of joint function caused by the disease can result in inactivity, further increasing osteoporosis risk. Studies also show that bone loss in rheumatoid arthritis may occur as a direct result of the disease.

The bone loss is most distinct in areas immediately surrounding the affected joints of concern. Which explains why women, a group already at increased risk for osteoporosis, are two to three times more likely to have rheumatoid arthritis as well.

LUPUS DICTIONARY

THE LUPUS DICTIONARY was formed to make it easier for you to have a chat with your physician or whom I recommend which is a naturopathic doctor or telling other people with lupus. It contains a list of lupus-related words and their meanings. Mainly focus on the most common type of lupus, systemic lupus erythematosus (SLE). If you have any questions about what rheumatology is or just want to stay updated, you can go online and research the American College of Rheumatology (ACR).

The American College of Rheumatology (ACR) is an international medical society representing over ninety-four hundred rheumatologists and rheumatology health professionals with a mission to empower rheumatology professionals to excel in their specialty. In doing so, the ACR offers education, research, advocacy, and practice management support to help its members continue their innovative work and provide quality patient care. Rheumatologists are experts in the diagnosis, management, and treatment of more than one hundred different types of arthritis and rheumatic diseases. However, so is naturopathic doctors so call them up.

Anemia: A condition in which the number of red blood cells, which carry oxygen throughout the body, is lower than normal. Anemia is common in patients with SLE.

Antibody: A type of molecule that circulates within the body. When antibodies are functioning correctly, they protect the body from foreign invaders, such as viruses and bacteria.

Antigen: A particle that causes the immune system to respond. Antigens can be foreign invaders such as viruses and bacteria. In patients with lupus, they can also be parts of the person's cells.

Antinuclear antibody (ANA): An antibody that binds to DNA and proteins contained within the cell nucleus. Patients with SLE typically have higher levels of ANA that people without lupus.

Arthralgia: Joint pain. Among patients with SLE, 80 percent experience this symptom at some point during the disease.

Arthritis: Inflammation of the joints. Arthritis can lead to joint pain (arthralgia) and reduced range of motion. Approximately 80 percent of patients with SLE experience pain caused by joint inflammation.

Autoantibody: An antibody that recognizes and destroys the body's cells. In SLE, autoantibodies attach to the body's healthy cells, which can cause inflammation and organ tissues.

B cell: A type of white blood cell that, as part of the immune system, produces antibodies that attach to foreign invaders.

Bacteria: Microscopic foreign invaders, such as salmonella, can cause infection.

Biopsy: The process of removing small tissue samples from a patient for examination. A biopsy may be performed to diagnose a disease or condition such as lupus nephritis (kidney inflammation caused by SLE).

Blood Chemistry: A test that measures levels of blood sugar, cholesterol elements, and different blood cells to help identify a variety of medical conditions.

Cardiologist: A physician who diagnoses and treats heart-related conditions.

Cardiovascular: Related to the heart and blood vessels. High blood pressure and other heart-related conditions can occur in people with SLE.

Carotid Plaque: Fatty material that lines the walls of the arteries that supply blood from the heart to the neck and head. Symptoms associated with carotid plaque vary in patients with SLE; however, patients with lupus typically experience carotid plaque disease symptoms at an earlier age than patients without lupus.

Cell: The smallest unit of living structure that can perform special functions. Patients with SLE may develop an immune response against some of their cells, causing them to be misidentified as foreign invaders.

Central Nervous System (CNS): The system that includes the brain and spinal cord. CNS symptoms of SLE include mood disorders, difficulty thinking, and seizures and vary from mild to severe. However, many common CNS symptoms can be side effects of certain medications or be caused by other medical conditions.

Chronic: Refers to a health condition lasting for a long time, typically more than three months. SLE is a chronic autoimmune disease.

Cognitive Impairment: Difficulty with thinking, learning, and memory. Cognitive impairment is one of many neurologic manifestation patients with SLE may experience.

Complement: A group of proteins in the blood that works with antibodies to help destroy bacteria and viruses, produce inflammation, and regulate immune reactions. Patients with SLE often have low complement levels, which may be associated with tissue inflammation and damage.

Complete Blood Count (CBC): A test used to determine the number of red blood cells, white blood cells, and platelets. A CBC may be performed to check for anemia or other abnormalities.

Coronary Heart Disease: Also known as coronary artery disease. Coronary heart disease is caused by a decrease in the blood flow from the arteries to the heart. Individuals with this condition usually have chest pain or heart damage. This disease affects many patients with SLE, especially younger women.

Cutaneous Lupus: A type of lupus affecting the skin. It is characterized by patchy areas on the face or other sun-exposed areas.

Depression: A temporary or chronic mental state associated with feelings of sadness, loneliness, low self-esteem, or reduced general daily function or interest in social interactions. Living with lupus may be challenging, and depression is common.

Dermatologist: A physician who diagnoses and treats skin-related conditions.

Discoid Rash: Skin irritation or redness that appears as a circular shape. Some patients with SLE may develop a discoid rash, characterized by the appearance of patchy, coin-shaped areas of skin on the face or other sun-exposed areas.

Disease Activity: Refers to the number of signs and symptoms and their severity.

Drug-induced Lupus: A type of lupus that is caused using certain drugs. Its symptoms are like those of SLE, and drug-induced lupus usually disappears if the drug is stopped.

Dysfunction: Impaired or abnormal function.

Edema: The presence of extra fluid between cells, tissues, or body cavities. Examples of edema include swelling of the feet, ankles, and legs, which can be symptoms of SLE associated with lupus nephritis.

Electrolyte: A particle in the bloodstream, including sodium, chloride, magnesium, and calcium.

Erythrocyte sedimentation rate (ESR): A blood test performed to identify general inflammation. An elevated ESR is commonly found in individuals with active SLE.

Fatigue: A lack of energy or weakness. Fatigue is the most commonly experienced symptom of SLE and may occur even when no other symptoms are present.

Fever: An increase in internal body temperature that occurs when the immune system is trying to protect and repair the body. More than 60 percent of patients with SLE experience occasional, temporary fever, typically caused by infection.

Flare: New or worsening disease activity. A sudden outburst of something, especially violence or a medical condition. Sun exposure and pregnancy may cause flares in patients with SLE.

Gastroenterologist: A physician who diagnoses and treats disorders of the digestive system.

Gastrointestinal: Related to the stomach and intestines. Many gastrointestinal problems are associated with, but not specific to, SLE, including symptoms such as dry mouth, nausea, and vomiting.

Genetic Disorder: A disease that is related to changes in a person's DNA and may be passed from a parent to a child. Although genetics is a contributing factor in the development of SLE, other factors may also cause the disease to develop.

Heart Attack: A sudden and sometimes fatal occurrence of coronary thrombosis, typically resulting in the death of part of a heart muscle.

Hematologic: Related to the blood or tissues that make blood. Patients with SLE may experience a wide range of blood disorders, such as low red blood cell count (anemia), low white blood cell count (leukopenia), or low platelet count (thrombocytopenia).

Hematologist: A physician who diagnoses and treats blood disorders.

Immune System: The system that consists of cells, tissues, and organs that work together to recognize and fight foreign invaders and help keep the body healthy. Foreign invaders include viruses, bacteria, parasites, and fungi. In patients with SLE, the immune system functions abnormally and attacks the body's tissue.

Immunologic Disorder: An impaired or abnormal functioning of the immune system.

Immunosuppressive: A medication capable of reducing the activity of the immune system.

Inflammation: The body's response after an injury or infection to repair and heal itself. Inflammation is commonly identified by redness, heat, swelling, and pain. In patients with SLE, inflammation may cause tissue damage over time.

Kidney: A major organ that removes waste products and maintains fluid and electrolyte balance. Kidney function is commonly affected in patients with SLE.

Leukopenia: A decrease in the number of white blood cells. This abnormality, which may occur in up to 20 percent of patients, can result from SLE and may become more severe because of disease flares or the use of immunosuppressive drugs.

Lupus: An inflammatory autoimmune disease that affects the functions of many different biological systems and occurs when the body creates antibodies that attack its own tissue. There are four types of lupus, one being systemic lupus erythematosus (SLE)

Lymphocyte: A type of white blood cell that circulates in the blood. Lymphocytes help the immune system protect the body from foreign invaders, such as bacteria, viruses, and infected or cancerous cells.

Lymphopenia: A condition in which levels of lymphocytes are lower than normal.

Macrophage: A type of cell that removes old cells and other unwanted material from the blood.

Malar rash: Skin irritation or redness on the cheeks. This type of rash, also known as a butterfly rash, extends over the cheeks and the bridge of the nose. A malar rash may range in severity from general redness to severe irritation. It can become more severe with exposure to sunlight.

Medical Examination: An examination of the body performed by a healthcare professional to diagnose, prevent, or cure a disease. This examination is completed as a preliminary assessment before the diagnosis of lupus or any other disease or condition is made.

Musculoskeletal: Related to the muscles and bones in the body. It is common for patients with SLE to experience conditions that affect the musculoskeletal system, such as arthritis.

Myalgia: Muscular pain, commonly in the arms and legs. In patients with SLE, myalgia is a sign of musculoskeletal system involvement.

Myocardial Infarction: Also known as a heart attack, this occurs when there is a lack of blood supply to a section of the heart for a long period of time. Patients with SLE, even below the age of thirty-five, may experience higher levels of heart attack than those without lupus.

Nephritis: Inflammation of the kidneys. Lupus nephritis is a serious kidney disorder caused by SLE.

Nephrologist: A physician who diagnoses and treats conditions that affect the kidneys.

Neurologic Disorder: An impaired or abnormal functioning of the nerves and muscles.

Ophthalmologist: A physician who diagnoses and treats conditions affecting the eyes.

Oral Ulcer: An ulcer of the mouth.

Organ: A part of the body that has a specific function, such as breathing air or digesting food. SLE may impact organs such as the lungs, heart, kidneys, and brain and can cause them not to function properly.

Pericarditis: Inflammation of the sac covering the heart. The cardiac abnormality is commonly observed in patients with SLE and is characterized by chest pain, shortness of breath, and abnormal fevers.

Photosensitivity: Increased sensitivity to sunlight; direct sunlight may cause a skin rash to form or become worse. Photosensitivity is common in Caucasian patients; however, all patients with SLE should avoid direct, prolonged exposure to the sun.

Platelet: A type of blood cell that helps the blood to clot following an injury.

Pleuritis: Inflammation of the inside lining of the chest space. Pleuritis is the most common respiratory manifestation of SLE.

Proteinuria: Presence of abnormally high levels of protein in the urine. Testing for protein in the urine may indicate whether a patient with SLE had kidney damage.

Psychosis: Abnormal functioning of the mind, characterized by loss of contact with reality and impairment of the cognitive processes.

Rash: An eruption of the skin on the body. SLE patients commonly develop a malar rash and may develop other types of skin rashes. Also, see discoid rash and malar rash.

Raynaud's Phenomenon: A condition caused by narrowing of blood vessels in the fingers and toes when exposed to extremely cold temperatures or stress. This condition causes the extremities to become cold and pale or bluish. A tingling sensation or pain may be experienced when normal circulation returns. Raynaud's phenomenon is common in patients with SLE, and symptoms can range from mild discomfort to the development of painful skin ulcers.

Remission: A lack of signs and symptoms.

Renal Disorder: A disturbance or decrease in kidney function resulting from disease. Renal damage is one of the most common and serious conditions caused by SLE, affecting half of all patients with lupus.

Rheumatologist: A physician who specializes in the study, diagnosis, and treatment of pain and conditions affecting the musculoskeletal system. A rheumatologist can determine whether a patient has SLE and can help manage the disease symptoms affecting the muscles and bones.

Seizure: A sudden onset of convulsions, loss of consciousness, or changes in the five senses due to abnormal electrical functions in the brain. SLE may cause seizures, which may affect up to 20 percent of patients.

Serositis: Inflammation of the tissues that surround parts of the body. Types of serositis include pleuritis and pericarditis, which are conditions associated with SLE.

Sign: An abnormality found when a physician does a physical exam or a lab test.

Symptom: An abnormal event or incident that is caused by a disease and reported by a patient to a physician. SLE is a unique disease because of the wide range of symptoms that patients may experience. Symptoms of lupus include headache or fatigue.

Systemic Lupus Erythematosus (SLE): A chronic autoimmune disease that can affect nearly every part of the body, including the skin, joints, lungs, heart, kidneys, brain, and blood. SLE is also commonly referred to as lupus.

T cell: A cell in the immune system responsible for recruiting other immune cells to protect the body against foreign invaders. In SLE, T cells do not function properly and contribute to the development of the disease.

Thrombocytopenia: An abnormally low number of platelets circulating in the blood. Platelets are needed to help the blood clot following an injury. Thrombocytopenia occurs in 25 to 35 percent of patients with SLE.

Tissue: A group of specialized cells that perform a specific in the body. In SLE, the body incorrectly identifies its own tissues as a foreign invader and signals the immune system to respond.

Titer: The amount of a substance, such as the level of antibodies in the blood. A screening test for ANAs is standard for assessing SLE. Patients with lupus typically have high titers of ANAs.

Ulcer: An inflamed wound on the skin or inner lining of parts of the body, such as in the mouth and nose, caused by loss of tissue. Ulcers may be caused by SLE or other diseases and conditions. In patients with lupus, sunlight may cause this form of irritation to occur on the skin.

Urinalysis: A test that analyzes urine and is used to diagnose kidney-related conditions. A healthcare professional may recommend this test to examine the health of the kidneys.

Virus: An agent that causes disease by infecting cells. A virus is a microscopic agent and is an example of a foreign invader that the immune system will try to destroy to protect the body.

White Blood Cell: A type of cell circulating in the blood that fights foreign invaders and is an important part of the body's immune defenses. Lymphocytes are one of the many different types of cells that can be classified as white blood cells. Certain conditions, such as SLE, can cause the level of white blood cells to be lower than normal.

X-ray: A test used to obtain images of bones, joints, and other dense tissues. This test may be recommended by a healthcare professional to determine the extent of organ involvement in disease.

> You only get one life, so I don't want to be known for one thing but for everything I do.
>
> —LaTonya Bias, PhD

End

> You are a victim of your health. No one will hit you harder than life itself, so stand tall and have a relationship between you and Lupus.
>
> —LaTonya Bias, PhD

One thing I want you to get out of this book is that time is precious, and despite my stories, I am sure you have one too. So spread the word about lupus. Become an advocate. Give this book to someone you think will enjoy it or who you want to learn firsthand about lupus and some history of me. I hope you enjoyed taking a walk through the life of autoimmune disease with me. To learn more about the next steps with lupus, please read part 2 *Does CBD & MARIJUANA Help Lupus*. This book is a great inspirational volume that will allow you to follow God on steps for never giving up. Flare-ups can destroy or take your life. It is all in how you handle the process.

REFERENCE

Gereda JE, Leung DYM, Thatayatikom A, Streib JE, Price MR, Klinnert MD, et al. Relationship between house dust endotoxin exposure, type 1 T-cell development, and allergen sensitization in infants at high risk of asthma. Lancet 2000; 355:1680–1683.

Jones CA, Holloway JA, Warner JO. Does atopic disease start in fetal life? Allergy 2000; 55:2–1

American Medical Association (AMA) information on advance directives website: http://www.arthritis.org

FDA Food Pyramid web site brochure: http://www.pueblo.gsa.gov.cic text/food-pyramid/main

Lupus Foundation of America articles: http://www.lupus.gor

National Institutes of Health and National Institute of Arthritis and Musculoskeletal and Skin Disease website: http://www.nih.gov

WebMD website, for reliable generalized medical information in abstracts and full article from: http://www.webmd.com

Dwight H. Kono & Argyrios N. Theofilopouuos (2009) Genetics of Systemic Autoimmunity in Mouse Models of Lupus, International Reviews of Immunology, 19:4-5, 367-387, DOI: 10.3109/0883018 0009055504

Dean, Gillian S., et al. "Cytokines and systemic lupus erythematosus." Ann Rheum Dis 2000; 59: 243–251.

"Systemic lupus erythematosus." In-Depth Patient Education Reports. Ed. Harvey Simon. 21 Jan. 2008. University of Maryland Medical Center. 25 June 2009 <http://www.umm.edu/patiented/articles/what_causes_systemic_lupus_erythematosus_000063_2.htm>.

Wallace, Daniel J. The Lupus Book: A Guide for Patients and Their Families. 1st ed. New York: Oxford University Press, 1995. Prescription for Nutritional Healing Fourth Edition Phyllis A. Balch.

CPSIA information can be obtained
at www.ICGtesting.com
Printed in the USA
BVHW072027010720
581819BV00001B/35